PSYCHOLOGY RESEARCH PROGRESS

A SOCIO-ECONOMIC AND DEMOGRAPHIC ANALYSIS OF MENTAL WELLBEING

THE INDIAN CASE

PSYCHOLOGY RESEARCH PROGRESS

Additional books and e-books in this series can be found on Nova's website under the Series tab.

PSYCHOLOGY RESEARCH PROGRESS

A SOCIO-ECONOMIC AND DEMOGRAPHIC ANALYSIS OF MENTAL WELLBEING

THE INDIAN CASE

ANTONIO RODRIGUEZ ANDRES
AND
SIDDHARTHA MITRA
EDITORS

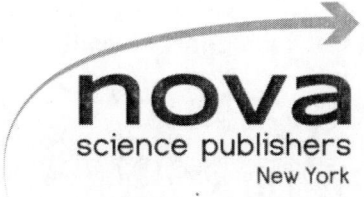

Copyright © 2021 by Nova Science Publishers, Inc.

All rights reserved. No part of this book may be reproduced, stored in a retrieval system or transmitted in any form or by any means: electronic, electrostatic, magnetic, tape, mechanical photocopying, recording or otherwise without the written permission of the Publisher.

We have partnered with Copyright Clearance Center to make it easy for you to obtain permissions to reuse content from this publication. Simply navigate to this publication's page on Nova's website and locate the "Get Permission" button below the title description. This button is linked directly to the title's permission page on copyright.com. Alternatively, you can visit copyright.com and search by title, ISBN, or ISSN.

For further questions about using the service on copyright.com, please contact:
Copyright Clearance Center
Phone: +1-(978) 750-8400   Fax: +1-(978) 750-4470   E-mail: info@copyright.com.

NOTICE TO THE READER

The Publisher has taken reasonable care in the preparation of this book, but makes no expressed or implied warranty of any kind and assumes no responsibility for any errors or omissions. No liability is assumed for incidental or consequential damages in connection with or arising out of information contained in this book. The Publisher shall not be liable for any special, consequential, or exemplary damages resulting, in whole or in part, from the readers' use of, or reliance upon, this material. Any parts of this book based on government reports are so indicated and copyright is claimed for those parts to the extent applicable to compilations of such works.

Independent verification should be sought for any data, advice or recommendations contained in this book. In addition, no responsibility is assumed by the Publisher for any injury and/or damage to persons or property arising from any methods, products, instructions, ideas or otherwise contained in this publication.

This publication is designed to provide accurate and authoritative information with regard to the subject matter covered herein. It is sold with the clear understanding that the Publisher is not engaged in rendering legal or any other professional services. If legal or any other expert assistance is required, the services of a competent person should be sought. FROM A DECLARATION OF PARTICIPANTS JOINTLY ADOPTED BY A COMMITTEE OF THE AMERICAN BAR ASSOCIATION AND A COMMITTEE OF PUBLISHERS.

Additional color graphics may be available in the e-book version of this book.

Library of Congress Cataloging-in-Publication Data

ISBN: 978-1-53619-023-6

Published by Nova Science Publishers, Inc. † New York

CONTENTS

Preface		vii
Chapter 1	Interaction among Socioeconomic, Institutional, and Genetic Correlates of Adult Mental Health: Evidence from a Representative Sample from Urban Kolkata, India *Piyali Dasgupta and Bidisha Chakraborty and Siddhartha Mitra*	1
Chapter 2	Suicide in India *David Lester, Bijou Yang and Kavita Naik*	27
Chapter 3	What Leads to Happiness among Chronically Ill Individuals? *Debangana Chakraborty and Anindita Chaudhuri*	39
Chapter 4	College Mental Health in India: Coping with a Potential Crisis *Rajlakshmi Guha*	57
Chapter 5	Examining the Happiness Stimulating impacts of Close Relationships *Samadrita Saha and Anindita Chaudhuri*	85

Chapter 6	Mental Health Scenario in India *Abhay Kumar De*	**105**
Chapter 7	The Male-Female Ratio of Suicide Rates as a Measure of Gender Bias *Siddhartha Mitra, Sangeeta Shroff* *and Vanshika Agarwal*	**135**

About the Editors — **161**

Index — **163**

PREFACE

A holistic study of the mental health problem in India is important as it is home to more than 17.5% of the world's population and still needs to grow economically at a fast pace, given that the incidence of poverty is high and per capita income low in spite of the rapid economic growth registered in the past three decades. A rapidly increasing incidence of mental illness and other cases of deficient mental well-being is not only hampering human capital formation but also the effectiveness of the stock of human capital that is already in place. In 2015-16, the National Mental Health Survey of India reported that an estimated 13.7 per cent of India's population suffered from one or the other kind of mental illness. There is ample evidence that this is the outcome of a worsening situation – consider the incidence of suicides in India which has leapfrogged from 6.3 per 100,000 in 1980 to 10.4 in 2019, as pointed out by authors contributing to this volume (Lester, Yang and Naik), an increase of more than 60% in about 4 decades. It is important to halt or reverse this alarming trend not only for economic reasons but to maximize the proportion of the population which is able to derive happiness and fulfilment from life, something which should be considered to be a human right.

This book represents, to the best of our knowledge, the first comprehensive study of the mental health problem in India as it looks at the problem from all angles – the causes and consequences, extreme manifestations such as the incidence of suicides, the plight of the vulnerable population groups such as the youth and those suffering from chronic illnesses, the measures that can be used to tackle the problem at the level of the individual and the policy maker etc. It also looks at what the incidence of mental health problems tells us about the magnitude of other problems facing society, such as gender bias.

Any such comprehensive approach obviously requires contributions from scholars hailing from different disciplines. This book is the outcome of contributions by economists (Vanshika Agarwal, Antonio Rodriguez Andres, Bidisha Chakraborty, Piyali Dasgupta, Bijou Yang, Siddhartha Mitra, Kavita Naik and Sangeeta Shroff in no order of importance), psychologists (Debangana Chakraborty, Anindita Chaudhuri, Rajlakshmi Guha, David Lester and Samadrita Saha again in no order of importance) and a psychiatrist (Abhay De). Where necessary an interdisciplinary approach has been adopted, such as the study on the probable causes and associates of suicides in India by Lester, Yang and Naik. The approach used by all authors is evidence based: primary surveys carried out by some of the authors, secondary data from reliable sources and a review of relevant literature. Standard techniques such as multivariate regression analysis and statistical correlation have been used to derive results, wherever possible, from data. In short, the 'scientific method' has been used.

In the rest of this chapter we try to sew the snapshots of the various chapters of this book into a general but multidimensional overview of the mental health problem in India. The reader should bear in mind that this overview is only rough and no substitute for the richness and depth of content in various chapters. We start from the twin contributions of Dasgupta, Chakraborty and Mitra; and Lester, Yang and Naik. In the first contribution the authors look at the incidence of self-reported wellbeing, a deficit of which may or may not be associated with mental illness and determining factors. The authors conclude through empirical analysis that poor well-being is an outcome of genetic, economic (such as unemployment and economic deprivation) and social factors (such as lack of safety of women) as well as poor physical health. Lester, Yang and

Naik's study bases its findings on All India and regional data on suicides which are predominantly the outcome of mental illness accompanied by triggers such as adverse socio-economic circumstances and life events. The study points to urbanization and low life expectancy as factors positively associated with suicide rates in populations. Urbanization pushing up suicide rates seems to indicate that enhanced stresses of life, often associated with urbanization, contribute to suicides. Low life expectancy, on the other hand, might be partially an outcome of high suicide rates or correlated with other factors such as poor physical health and socio-economic and physical security (as noted by Dasgupta, Chakraborty and Mitra) which contribute to an elevation of the suicide rate through diminished mental well-being. Lester et al. also seem to indicate that culture and lifestyle, often the outcome of the religion practiced, is a significant determinant of suicide – they find that populations with a higher percentage of Muslims have lower suicide rates.

Two of the contributions – the first by Debangana Chakraborty and Anindita Chaudhuri and the second by Rajlakshmi Guha – draw our attention to vulnerable groups: those who are chronically ill and the college going youth of the country. The first group has to wage a lifelong battle with the physical burden imposed by illnesses such as diabetes and coronary heart disease. Youth entering college have to deal with the challenges of evolving brain chemistry and structure and changing life circumstances, which include greater autonomy and responsibilities and romantic relationships as well as make or break competition. Chakraborty and Chaudhuri highlight the importance of coping with chronic illness and point to the positive role that emotional intelligence (regulation of emotional reactions to the expressed emotions of other human beings as well as life circumstances such as the physical burden and pain imposed by disease) and lifestyle practices such as meditation and yoga can play in this regard. Guha points to the alarming increase in the incidence of mental health disorders – anxiety disorders, depression, disorders caused by substance abuse and others – among college going students in India. She emphasizes the need for universalizing sensitization and awareness programs in regard to mental health at the level of the college as well as counselling centers that work in liaison with academic units within institutions. She also recognizes that the problems confronting the youth and their psychological ramifications are an outcome of culture and academic environment and yet a function of time. This implies that policy makers should from time to time revise their approach to tackling the problem of mental illness among college students.

The two contributions mentioned immediately above provide for some measures at the level of the individual or policy makers for curbing and managing the incidence of mental illness and stimulating mental well-being. The research by Samadrita Saha and Anindita Chaudhuri provides an invaluable supplement to these studies by looking at the happiness stimulating impacts of close relationships and providing empirical evidence for the significance of such impact mediated through empathy, positivity and strong emotional bonds.

The contributions discussed till now have not looked at the national architecture of policies, laws and institutions for dealing with the problem of deficient mental health in the country. A review of recent developments by Abhay De reveals significant positives: a national mental health policy, a rights-based mental health act and a mental health programme which attempts to link service at the doorstep of every household to the network of primary and community health centres, mental hospitals and nodal centres. Yet major problems remain, primarily those arising from paucity of skilled manpower and the long distances often separating the household and quality medical care.

The last contribution by Siddhartha Mitra, Sangeeta Shroff and Vanshika Agarwal is different from the others as it uses data on suicides, an outcome of mental illness and various triggers, to throw light on a separate but linked problem, that of gender bias in society. Here there is good news: 80% of the states and union territories have shown a significant growth in the ratio of male and female suicide rates over roughly the last three decades, thus pointing to an improvement in the status of women in most of the country. It also concludes on the basis of empirical analysis that an improvement in overall literacy is a powerful mechanism to reduce gender bias as revealed by the mentioned ratio: education makes women more aware of their rights and men more enlightened.

To conclude, as editors we consider ourselves fortunate to present a book consisting of pioneering contributions from scholars who highlight different but related aspects of the mental health problem in India. We are hopeful that this will stimulate more multidisciplinary as well as interdisciplinary research in this area that is of use to the society in general as well as policy makers.

Antonio Rodríguez Andrés
Siddhartha Mitra

In: A Socio-Economic and Demographic ... ISBN: 978-1-53619-023-6
Editors: A. Rodriguez Andres et al. © 2021 Nova Science Publishers, Inc.

Chapter 1

INTERACTION AMONG SOCIOECONOMIC, INSTITUTIONAL, AND GENETIC CORRELATES OF ADULT MENTAL HEALTH: EVIDENCE FROM A REPRESENTATIVE SAMPLE FROM URBAN KOLKATA, INDIA

Piyali Dasgupta[1], and Bidisha Chakraborty[2]
and Siddhartha Mitra[2]*

[1]Sarsuna College, affiliated under Calcutta University, Kolkata, India
[2]Jadavpur University, Kolkata, India

ABSTRACT

According to the latest WHO report on depression and National Mental Health Survey of India for 2015 – 2016, over a 100 million Indians suffer from mental health problems requiring expert intervention,

---

* Corresponding Author's E-mail: pdg2009@rediffmail.com.

with a majority living in urban areas. The associated huge loss of human resources results in sub-optimal productivity and economic performance, and hence loss of social welfare. In this context, we try to identify individual characteristics which result in proneness to mental ill-health and measures to blunt the effect of these characteristics and promote mental health. This is done by administering a questionnaire for measuring mental health, based on previous such questionnaires in the literature, to a random sample of 500 Indian adults, residing in a Kolkata municipal ward between 2014 and 2015, to generate relevant data for estimation of an ordered probit model. The results highlight that both genetic and socio-economic characteristics - family history of suicide, unemployment (voluntary and involuntary), poor physical health, long term disease, digestive disorders, tragic life events and alcohol disorders - are significantly related to mental health of individuals. The study reveals that some protection from mental illness can be achieved through policy enabled augmentation of family income involving creation of physical assets and provision of opportunities for employment and better education, better local governance, facilitation of greater political freedom, enhancement of safety of women, and promotion of sound physical health through awareness generation and preventive and curative measures.

Keywords: socio-economic indicators, institutional factors, genetic factors, physical health, diseases, ordered probit, mental health, urban India

INTRODUCTION

According to the report of the National Mental Health Survey of India, 2015 -2016, "every sixth Indian needs mental health help; urban areas are the most affected; at least 13.7 per cent of India's general population has been projected to be suffering from a variety of mental illnesses; and 10.6 percent of these requires immediate intervention". These findings are consistent with those of the latest WHO report on depression released in 2017, which says that almost 7.5% of Indians suffer from major or minor mental health problems requiring clinical treatment.

Mental health, an 'indivisible part of general health', is a major determinant of individual capability, effectiveness of human capital formation and social wellbeing. While casual empiricism reveals that educated and trained individuals suffer a significant and often drastic decrease in productivity due to sudden onset of mental illness, such losses have not been accurately measured. There continues to be a lack of appreciation of the need for promotion of mental health, especially the significance of determining socioeconomic factors which can be influenced through policy changes. Though our appreciation of genetic influences on human behavior and wellbeing has improved greatly in recent times, the scientific means available at our disposal for altering these effects are both inadequate and unavailable for use due to cultural and ethical reasons. At the same time the true impact of the socio-economic factors can be identified only if we control for the influence of genetic factors. Thus, this timely study assumes great importance as it provides recommendations for enhancing the level of mental wellbeing in a society after accounting for both socio-economic and genetic influences on such wellbeing.

As mentioned, this paper attempts a holistic examination of factors which affect mental health in India. The study cuts across disciplinary barriers to examine how socio-economic and institutional determinants, physical wellbeing and genetic factors affect mental health. The contribution of this paper lies not only in the mentioned holistic examination but also in yielding a picture of the interaction between a) factors that put an individual at risk of being afflicted by mental illness and b) protective measures, which yields valuable policy lessons.

The existing literature on mental health in India primarily focuses on the aggregate prevalence of mental morbidity (Dube, 1970; Nandi et al., 1986; Murthy, 1987a; Reddy et al., 1994; Ganguli, 2000); and its disaggregation on the basis of age, gender, sex and educational attainment (Verghese et al., 1973), occupation (Dube, 1970; Verghese et al., 1973), income (Mueser and McGurk, 2004), poverty (Patel et al. , 2003), religion, migration (Dube, 1970; Nandi et al., 1992; Bhugra, 2004), marital status, caste and family type (Verghese et al., 1973). The relationship between low socio-economic status and mental health has received considerable attention in the recent literature on India (Patel et al., 1999; Das et al., 2007; Das et al., 2009; Das et al., 2012; Vijayakumar, 2007; Andrés et al.,

2014). However, these studies rely on proxy indicators of mental health e.g., suicide rates, hospitalization rates, use of health resources. This data obviously suffers from underreporting because of the stigma attached to mental illness in India and generates underestimates of population-wide psychiatric morbidity (Tannenbaum et al., 2009).

Empirical findings from existing literature suggest that the risk of developing mental health disorders is linked to variables such as income (Easterlin, 1995; Blanchflower and Oswald, 2002; Lakshmanasamy, 2010), type of employment or unemployment (Goldsmith et al., 1996; Avery et al., 2004; Di Tella et al., 2001; Whelan, 1992; Artazcoz, 2004), occupational stress (Choi et al., 2008), debt (Richardson et al., 2013), overall health (Graham, 2008; Raphael et al., 2005; Patten, 1999), chronic physical conditions and long term diseases (Robson and Gray, 2007; Himelhoch et al., 2004; Grigsby et al., 2002), substance abuse (Phillips and Johnson, 2001), education (Cutler et al., 2006; Korten and Henderson, 2000), parenthood (Evenson and Simon, 2005; Stanca, 2012), migration (Bhugra and Jones, 2001), quality of governance and the size of social capital (Helliwell, 2003), political, economic and private freedoms (Veenhoven, 2000), and life events (Simon, 2002; Wheaton,1990).

Unlike most previous studies which ascertain the lack of mental health on the basis of detected morbidity, we measure the impact of various socioeconomic factors affecting mental health. We measure mental health on the basis of individual perceptions of wellbeing. These are observed on a calibrated scale that allows us to account for the deficiency of mental health a) associated with mental illness as well as b) lack of wellbeing not manifested in mental illness. To the extent, that category a) is a more extreme form of deficiency than that in b), our study helps us to determine the direction and intensity of the impact of various socioeconomic factors on mental wellbeing more accurately. Further, individuals often end up in category a) by transitioning through category b). Thus, the measured impacts would help generate important policies regarding employment generation and education and a host of other influences that would prevent people from falling into categories a) and b) from states of good mental health or help those in category b) to move out of it by improving their mental health instead of stagnating in regard to their wellbeing or moving into category a).

In our study we have used a mental health questionnaire, based on a study of previous questionnaire in the literature, for determining the association between mental health and different socioeconomic correlates. It is to be noted that most of the previous users of such questionnaires (e.g., Patel et al., 2008; Endsley et al., 2017; Singh and Kashyap, 2016) have concentrated on the examination of psychometric properties, reliability and validity of tools for measuring mental health status. Thus, our study fills an important gap in the literature.

MODELLING APPROACHES: THEORETICAL UNDERPINNINGS

Following Dalgard (2008), Lincoln et al. (2003), and Umberson (1993), we assume that the mental health of an individual is affected by family income and background; physical health outcomes including various ends of morbidity; social connections measured by number of friends and membership of networks; selective institutional factors such as perceived quality of governance , safety of women, political freedom and caste based discrimination; and stress and competition as well as pollution caused by urbanization.

Intuitively, family income and the value of physical assets should exhibit very high positive association. The same should be true for education and the type of employment, especially in the sample that we have studied. Therefore, our single equation regression model includes one variable from each of these two pairs of variables to avoid multicollinearity problems. The familial characteristics which are considered are prevalence of family discord; family structure as revealed by the 'joint' or 'nuclear' nature of a family, and family size.

Family discord can stem from inadequate absolute level of family income, lower family income relative to that of neighbors, indebtedness etc. Marital discord can arise due to incompatibility between husband and wife, often observed in a newlywed couple because of a lack of chemistry or in an aged couple due to disaffection and pressures and tensions at the workplace; substance abuse by family members including alcoholism; and life events such as birth of a close one, death of a close one and end of a relationship.

It is a common perception among psychiatrists that mental illnesses "run in the family" (The Centre for Genetics Education, 2012). Mukherjee (2016) opines that these results when genetic predispositions are triggered by adverse environmental conditions. The negative effect of such genetic predispositions is captured in our study by ascertaining whether there is an ancestral history of depression or suicide.

Finally, we form the mental health function, in which we consider the mental health score as an ordinal variable which depends on the above mentioned independent variables. An ordered probit model is used to estimate this function. We assume that the error term in the model measures the unobserved heterogeneity (e.g., individual characteristics such as attitudinal factors impacting mental health) that are not captured in our data and follows a standard normal distribution. We use exclusion restrictions by choosing different sets of explanatory variables in the equations. The impact of an explanatory variable on the dependent variable is measured through the estimation of marginal effects.

OUR MENTAL HEALTH MEASURE

We use a questionnaire based on previous questionnaires in the literature to assess mental health status. The questionnaire has been constructed so that it only generates reliable data on variables related to mental health. The tool derived from this questionnaire can be seen clearly to be measuring mental health and is unaffected by measurement error and free of response bias. The assessed psychometric deficiencies of the individuals broadly belong to two classes: inability to carry out usual daily tasks, and the occurrence of new and distressing symptoms which significantly alter the individual's mental state. Each of the twelve questions in the questionnaire can be answered by choosing one out of 4 options. By choosing the first two options the individual places himself in the fairly or highly free stress category in regard to the aspect being investigated and gets a score of 1; the other choices correspond to stressed states and fetch him a score of zero. Thus, a dichotomous scoring method is adopted for each question and a final mental health score, ranging from 0 to 12, is obtained by adding up the scores across questions. Division by 12 results in a score between 0 and 1, the average aggregate score. The level of mental health is considered as being increasing in this aggregate score.

DATA

We collected primary data for 2014 and 2015 from *Municipality Ward 127* in Kolkata, a major metropolis located in Eastern India. The selection of an urban area for the survey can be justified on the grounds that urban areas show a higher incidence of mental ill health than rural areas (Harpham, 1994; Srivastava, 2009; Andrés et al., 2014). Further, urban areas such as Kolkata have been subjected to rapid changes in the recent past such as the fast-paced development of infrastructure exemplified by the Metrorail, hospitals, colleges and a significant influx of migrants. Such changes are often mentally destabilizing and disturbing.

The data were collected through a combination of face-to-face interviews, with permission taken from interviewees for academic use of collected data and assurance being given about preservation of anonymity. Out of the total adult population of 15,000, a sample of 600 units was drawn using a random sampling technique. The voter list of the studied ward provided information such as name, address, and age of those who are eligible to vote. Since a random and representative sample was drawn from this population, it reflected the socio-economic heterogeneity of the population.

In the process of data collection suitable explanations were provided in the local language to facilitate proper comprehension of questions, with emphasis laid on catalyzing a friendly atmosphere to improve compliance by respondents and data quality. Out of the 600 individuals originally targeted for sampling, 522 (or 87 percent) actually participated in the interview. However, the usable sample size was only about 500 as some respondents did not furnish the entire required information. Non-respondents were mostly middle aged. All necessary prior approvals needed for a survey of this kind were sought and given.

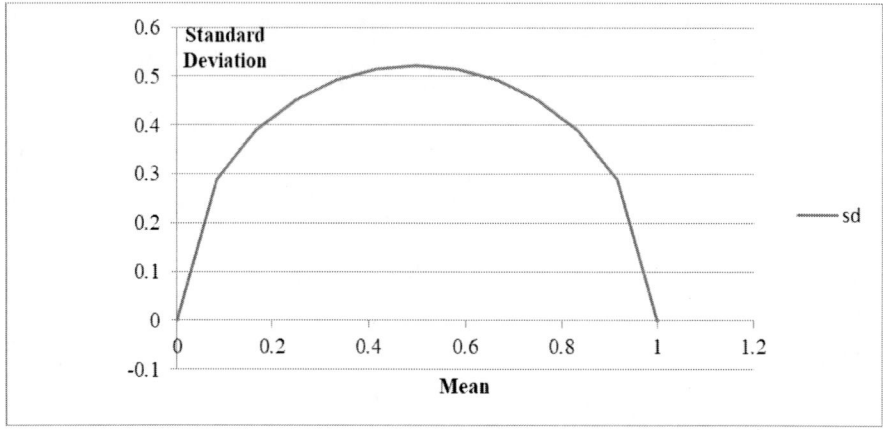

Figure 1. Relationship of standard deviation with mean for individual level question wise scores.

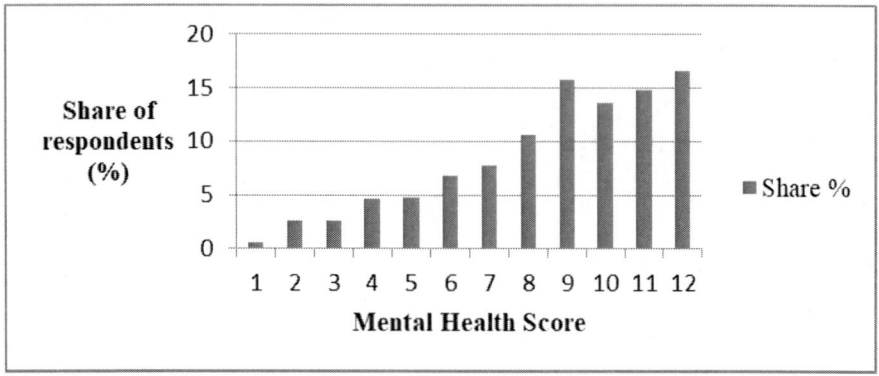

Figure 2. Distribution of the mental health scores.

We have calculated summary statistics such as the individual level mean and standard deviation of question wise scores. The graph between the standard deviation and the mean exhibits an inverted U-shaped relationship with the standard deviation maximized when mean is 0.5.

The distribution of mental health is shown in Figure 2. Roughly 17 percent of the respondents report that they are completely mentally healthy (a perfect aggregate score of 12) and 4.8 percent report a score of 3 or less, thus pointing to their suffering from a mental disorder. A study[1] conducted by the National Commission on Macroeconomics and Health in 2005 reported that nearly 5 percent of India's population suffer from common mental disorders such as depression and anxiety. Therefore, our result supports the finding from that study. We find that the mental health scores of only about 60 percent of the respondents are above or equal to 9, the lowest score associated with good mental health. It should be noted, however, that the distribution of mental health scores might have been different if the sample used for this study had included urban slum dwellers who had recently migrated from rural areas, children and adolescents aged below 18 years, as well as those who abstained from participation in the study.

The respondents are subdivided into five categories on the basis of family income: poor (24.6%), lower middle income (36%), middle income (24.2%),

upper middle income (11.6%) and rich (3.6%). Age, physical assets and education are considered as categorical variables by assigning numbers. We use dummy variables for measuring occupation (e.g., full time, unemployment), nature of job (e.g., permanent), sector wise job (e.g., public and organized), perceived health, self-reported diseases etc. We find that according to the data collected, 53.4% of respondents suffered from digestive disorders, 12% had a history of suicides in their family and 63.4% suffered from anxiety disorder. The variables are described in the Appendix (Table 1).

---

[1] Available at http://healthminds.in/blog/mental-illness-overview-status-in-india/.

RESULTS

The ordered probit regression result reveals that an increase in family income is likely to enhance mental health (see Appendix, Table 3, column 1-4). The finding for family income is in accordance with earlier studies such as Blanchflower and Oswald (2002); Easterlin (1995); Frey and Stutzer (2002); Di Tella, MacCulloch, and Oswald (2006); and Lakshmanasamy (2010). It is quite expected that enhancement of family income up to a certain level improves the living environment and material standard of living as well as access to health care services.

Furthermore, fulltime employment is seen to contribute positively to mental health, as compared to the other states corresponding to some lack of employment (voluntary and involuntary unemployment). This result is also in line with findings mentioned above (e.g., Clark and Oswald, 1994; Andrés et al., 2014) as well as the study by Rosenthal et al. (2012) who conclude on the basis of data that those employed full-time report the lowest psychological damage as well as stress and depression. The marginal effects of part-time employment, voluntary unemployment and involuntary unemployment starting from the base of full-time employment on mental health are negative in ascending order of magnitude (Table 3, column 4 and 5).

We find that the female proportion in the sample that reports itself as being voluntarily unemployed is 98.3%. On the other hand, there is very little voluntary unemployment among men. This can easily be explained on the basis of traditional attitudes within the society and family which consider the male householder to be the bread winner and the woman to be the homemaker. The shedding of such traditional attitudes and encouragement of women to aspire for work outside the family even after marriage is possible through suitable education, especially through various forms of media such as print and broadcasting. This should result in a significant improvement in mental health.

Note that (see Table 3, Column 1–3) respondents having poor physical health as well as displaying chronic anxiety are likely to have lower levels of mental health than others, ceteris paribus. Again, digestive disorders and long- term diseases are likely to lower mental health. The magnitudes of the estimated coefficients of chronic anxiety are much smaller than the coefficients for the other three mentioned factors.

Permanent workers (see Table 4) are likely to report better mental health as compared to temporary workers. Again, monthly salaried workers and the self – employed are likely to have better mental health than casual workers. Similarly, workers in the organized sector are seen to report higher mental health scores than those in the unorganized sector. The differences in mental health across different occupations can be apparently explained by the differences in terms and conditions such as work-life balance, job-security, flexibility in leave rules, work environment etc. Education is seen as likely to improve mental health (Table 3, column 1). Previous studies (e.g., Andres et al., 2014) that measured education either through the literacy rate or gross enrolment ratio had generated similar results.

Let us summarize results regarding the other control variables (in Table 4, Columns 1–5). Age has a negative effect on mental health as also found by Firdaus (2017) in the Indian context. Bohra et al. (2015) reported that depression is widely prevalent in women due to inadequate number of mental health professionals, lack of awareness, stigma, disadvantaged position of women, multiple roles, increased levels of stress, and domestic violence. Our study also shows that females are more likely to suffer from mental health problems. We also find that the respondents belonging to the minorities are more likely to have lower mental health. These findings indicate that wellbeing diminishing gender discrimination and discrimination against minorities are still widely prevalent in India.

Table 3 (columns 1–4) captures results regarding the effects of the perceptions of the survey respondents about their own condition, as revealed by different variables, measured on a four-point Likert scale. Respondents who are satisfied with the present level of absolute family income are seen to have better mental health. Greater sensitivity to relative income significantly lowers mental health. Economic freedom significantly improves mental health, leading to higher quality of life as it is positively associated with high productivity, low poverty, consequent improvement in living environments etc. There exists a direct relationship between good governance and mental health. Spiritual dependence (understood by the respondents as belief in God) significantly enhances mental health possibly by encouraging the formation of more positive attitudes. A similar result was found by Singh and Modi (2011).

Adverse life events, such as the end of a relationship and the death of a close one, have a significant adverse effect on mental health (Table 3 and Table 4). A similar finding has been reported by Ballas and Dorling (2007) regarding the end of relationships.

Mental health problems are more common among those who have a family history of suicide (Table 4) or depression (Table 3). This finding somewhat confirms previously emphasized genetic influence on mental health outcomes. The positively significant impact of political freedom and safety of women (Table 4) supports the view that participation in democracy generates positive effects on mental health (Layard, 2005; Frey and Stutzer, 2002) because of a seeming preference for democracy among humans. Similarly, the incidence of crimes against women has an adverse effect on mental health (for similar results see Andrés et al., 2014). Note that 2.5 million cases of crimes against women have been reported in India over the last decade; the share of the state of West Bengal – whose capital is Kolkata, the city in which this study has been conducted – was 9.6 per cent in 2016, far in excess of its population share[2].

Again, substantial reduction in financial stress, inflation, and surrounding poverty; work related anxiety and pressure; alcohol disorders; competition stress and pollution in urban areas; span of emigration; and family discord are also seen to affect mental health significantly. To make it easier to read the results from the ordered probit models, we report the marginal effects of the independent variables on the probability of being completely mentally healthy (this corresponds to achieving the maximum mental health score).

---

[2] NCRB data 2016.

DISCUSSION AND CONCLUSION

We have examined the predictors of mental health and find that unemployment (voluntary and involuntary), poor physical health, long term disease, digestive disorders, and history of suicide in family, life events and alcohol disorder put mental health at significant risk. On the other hand, higher family income and value of physical assets owned, greater education, generation of jobs in the public as well as organized sector, more economic and political freedom, good governance, cultivation of spirituality and enhanced safety of women are associated with better mental health outcomes.

Apart from generating an insight into the diverse socioeconomic and genetic determinants of mental health, these findings lead to obvious policy prescriptions such as awareness creation programmes to emphasize the connection between physical health and mental health; and generation of consciousness regarding genetic influences on mental health and provision of preventive and precautionary care for those who have a family history of depression and suicide; as well as creation of awareness regarding the negative impact of excessive consumption of alcohol on mental health. This is important as India is the world leader in regard to the annual number of suicides at the level of a nation according to data for 2013.

The population policy of India should also be reexamined with a view towards reformulation and changes in implementation in order to catalyze a reduction in the average family size. This would have positive implications for per capita income, the incidence of unemployment and inflation, all three of which impact mental wellbeing. Our findings also suggest that investment in social infrastructure and improvement in local governance, with emphasis on developing backward regions, might also be helpful.

The potential limitations of the data used in this study should be noted so as to inform future studies in the same research area. First, self-reported measures of mental health are often challenged based on reliability and validity (Bertrand and Mullainathan, 2001).

Secondly, this kind of data is associated with a difficulty in undertaking interpersonal comparisons of utility. Third, there could be some tendency for respondents to understate depression history, suicide history and alcohol intake because of stigma attached to mental illness and substance use disorder.

It should be noted though that respondents were assured that their identities would not be revealed after the survey, thus reducing this source of bias. Fourth, there is a problem of endogeneity.

For instance, it is reasonable to argue that those who suffer from poor mental health tend to be unemployed and this might account largely for the perceived causation running from unemployment to poor mental health. Nevertheless, the second type of causation might be weak. A similar argument can be made for education. There seems to be no easy way to resolve this issue of endogeneity. Fifth, since the data is cross-sectional, it is harder to establish the direction of causality.

Time and cost constraints have led to the use of a small sample which limits generalizability. For larger samples results could be different. Two standard methods, the instrumental variables approach and, alternatively, a long panel, are not feasible in this case.

The first is not feasible because it is difficult to find appropriate instruments of employment which are independent of mental health outcomes and the second because the study, carried out over a short time span and with limited funds, did not enable the collection of data from the same household at different points of time.

In spite of its weaknesses, our paper contributes to the literature, because we provide more evidence on the relationship between mental health and its socioeconomic, institutional and genetic correlates as we account for all degrees of deficiency in mental wellbeing, not just those which lead to incidence of mental illness. This is done through the pioneering combination of measuring psychological wellbeing through questionnaires and using sophisticated econometric tools to gain insight regarding the determinants of mental health.

APPENDIX

Table 1. Definitions and descriptive statistics of variables

Variable	Average (Standard Deviation)	Definition/measurement
Mental health	8.73 (2.69)	General health questionnaire is used to assess mental health assigning numbers 0, 1,…,12; highest mental health score = 12 and lowest mental health score = 0
Gender	0.52 (0.50)	Male = 1, Female = 0
Age	2.48 (0.79)	Age (years) is subdivided into four sub-groups assigning numbers such as 18 to 24years = 1; 25 to 44years = 2; 45 to 60years = 3; more than 61years = 4
Marital status	1.19 (0.39)	Married = 1 and Single = 0
Family income	2.35 (1.10)	Family income per month: less than Rs.5 000 = 1; Rs. 5 000 and less than Rs. 12 000 = 2; Rs.12 000 and less than Rs.30, 000 = 3; Rs. 30, 000 and less than Rs.60 000 = 4; Rs. 60, 000 and above = 5
Financial stress	1.62 (0.49)	Bear any kind of loan/ financial burden = 1, or zero otherwise
Physical Asset	3.80 (1.20)	Regular use of Radio, Gas Oven, T.V, Refrigerator, Air conditioner and Car, measured by assigning numbers as 1,…, 6 and otherwise zero so that more items indicate more physical asset
Employed full-time	0.37 (0.48)	Work for eight hours and half in a day and forty-eight hours in a week = 1 or zero otherwise
Employed part-time	0.21 (0.41)	Work for five to six hours in a day and thirty- six hours in a week = 1 or zero otherwise
Involuntary unemployed	0.05 (0.23)	Remain jobless after serious search of job for last three months or retrenched from the previous job = 1 or zero otherwise
Voluntarily unemployed	0.23 (0.42)	Not searching for job for last three months and age is less than or equal to sixty years = 1 or zero otherwise
Retired	0.11 (0.31)	Retired from service and age is more than sixty years = 1 or zero otherwise
Monthly Salaried	0.34 (0.48)	Earn fixed Salary per month = 1 or zero otherwise
Self Employed	0.19 (0.39)	Have own business = 1 or zero otherwise.
Public sector	0.12 (0.32)	Work in the government sector = 1 or zero otherwise

Table 1. (Continued).

Variable	Average (Standard Deviation)	Definition/ measurement
Organized sector	0.27 (0.44)	It does not include service workers such as midwives, domestic workers, barbers, vegetable and fruit vendors, newspaper vendors, pavement vendors, hand cart operator, etc.) = 1 or zero otherwise
Permanent job	0.86 (0.87)	No insecurity of losing the job) = 1 or zero otherwise
Education	3.78 (1.48)	Illiterate = 1, Primary = 2, Secondary = 3, Higher secondary = 4, Graduation = 5, Post-graduation/ PhD = 6
Post-Graduation	0.11 (0.32)	Completed Post graduation = 1 or zero otherwise.
Nuclear Family	1.51 (0.84)	Nuclear family = 1 and Joint Family = 0
Length of married life	17.31 (15.18)	Measured by number of years
Number of child = 1	0.37 (0.48)	Have one child = 1, zero otherwise
Number of child = 2	0.25 (0.43)	Have two children = 1, zero otherwise
Number of child >or = 3	0.09 (0.29)	Have three or more than three children = 1, zero otherwise
Family size	3.96 (1.75)	Indicated by number of members in the family
Span of immigration	24.55 (16.35)	Number of years immigrated from the rural area
Poor physical health	0.13 (0.34)	Perceived Physical health as poor = 1 or zero otherwise
Long term disease	0.12 (0.32)	Suffering from chronic disease (e.g., diabetes, arthritis, high blood pressure, heart diseases) = 1 or zero otherwise
Digestive disorder	0.53 (0.49)	Have common digestive problem (e.g., heartburn, diarrhea, gas, stomach pain etc.) = 1 or zero otherwise
Chronic anxiety	1.37 (0.48)	have excessive tension / worry about health, money, work, relationship etc. or have fear about everyday life events with no obvious reasons for worry: Yes = 1 or zero otherwise
Suicide history in family	0.12 (0.32)	Anyone from paternal or maternal side (not any one from in-laws) committed suicide = 1 zero otherwise
Alcohol disorder	0.28 (0.45)	Assertive self-report on the regular or occasional intake of alcohol = 1, or zero otherwise.
Minority caste	1.79 (0.40)	Belong to Schedule castes/ schedule tribe/ Muslims: Yes = 1 or zero otherwise
Social networking	0.35 (0.48)	Member of self-help group/ club/ organization/ face book etc. = 1 or zero otherwise

Variable	Average (Standard Deviation)	Definition/ measurement
Number of friends	7.28 (10.52)	Measured in numbers
Good governance	2.04 (0.63)	Self-assessment on the facilities and services provided by the local political body is rated as good = 1 or zero otherwise
Birth of close one	0.69 (0.46)	Recent personal experience (s) of having a baby in the family = 1or zero otherwise
Deaths of close one	0.63 (0.48)	Experiencing Death of a family member or close friend = 1 or zero otherwise
End of relationship	0.21 (0.41)	Recent personal Experience of end of a relationship e.g., separation, divorce, premarital break-up, widowhood and separation from children = 1or zero otherwise
Absolute income	2.57 (1.29)	Satisfied with the present level of the family income #
Relative income	1.95 (1.23)	Dissatisfaction related to lower income than most of friends, neighbors, and/or fellow workers #
Work anxiety	1.91 (1.25)	have fear of danger relating to job loss#
Work pressure	2.81 (1.20)	most days at work are quite stressful #
Wealth	2.22 (1.31)	Self-assessment regarding enhancement of satisfaction level by accrual of wealth (more money, jewelry, land ownership etc.) #
Inflation	3.19 (1.04)	Dissatisfaction arising out of the present inflationary situation #
Absence of poverty	3.45 (0.92)	Unhappiness arises from surrounding poverty #
Economic freedom	3.15 (1.16)	Have full control over own earning/ property #
Polluted environment	1.91(1.19)	Work/Live in a polluted environment #
Spiritual dependence	3.22 (1.15)	Self-assessment on spiritual dependence or believe in God as an essential for peaceful life#
Depression history	2.25 (1.28)	any family member remains in general depressed #
Stress-free atmosphere of urban area	2.13 (1.34)	Self-assessment on enhancement of happiness by avoiding the competition and stress

Answer is chosen out of 4 options (RensisLikert, 1931) - strongly disagree to strongly agree.

Table 2. Interim covariance and Cronbach's α

Cronbach's α	Total
Average interim covariance	0.037
Scale of reliability coefficient	0.747
Number of items in the scale	12

Table 3. Results from ordered probit models for mental health (Dummy for the maximum mental health level)

Explanatory Variables	Model 1	Model 2	Model 3	Model 4
Family income	0.021 (2.08)**	0.031 (3.31)***	0.033 (3.61)***	0.065 (6.19)***
Employed fulltime	-	0.079 (3.65)***	-	-
Employed part-time	-	-	- 0.024 (1.19)	- 0.050 (2.27)**
Involuntary unemployment	-	-	-0.083 (4.98)***	- 0.097 (4.84)***
Voluntary unemployment	-	-	-0.075 (4.24)***	-0.110 (6.00)***
Retired	-	-	-0.056 (2.71)***	-0.089 (4.44)***
Education	0.022(3.10)***	-	-	-
Poor physical health	-0.096 (6.32)***	-0.095 (6.28)***	-0.094 (6.16)***	-
Chronic anxiety	-0.06 (2.81)***	-0.065 (3.05)***	-0.059 (2.79)***	-
Good governance	0.069 (2.36)**	0.058 (2.08)**	0.056 (2.04)**	0.056 (1.83)*
End of relationship	-0.059 (3.56)***	-0.06 (3.80)***	-0.062 (3.80)***	-0.087 (4.78)***
Birth of a close one	-0.03 (1.65)*	-0.045 (2.20)**	-0.042 (2.06)**	-0.062 (4.78)***
Absolute income	0.016 (2.13)**	0.020 (2.52)**	0.023 (2.83)***	-
Relative income	-0.016 (2.12)**	-0.015 (2.07)**	-0.017 (2.27)***	-
Economic freedom	0.018 (2.46)***	0.018 (2.46)***	0.014 (1.88)*	-
Polluted environment	-0.028 (3.66)***	-0.027 (3.67)***	-0.028 (3.71)***	-
Spiritual dependence	0.015 (2.11)**	0.014 (1.95)**	0.016 (2.19)**	0.019 (2.25)**
Depression history	-0.03 (3.65)***	-0.025 (3.59)***	-0.026 (3.71)***	-0.035 (4.23)***
Family discord	-	-	-	-0.025 (2.91)***
Nuclear family	-	-	-	-0.006 (0.26)
Family size	-	-	-	-0.008 (1.41)
Y = Pr (mental health score = 12) =	0.104	0.102	0.101	0.123

Notes: Robust z statistics in parentheses.

*Significant at 10%; **significant at 5%; ***significant at 1%. The reported probit results are marginal effects.

Table 4. Results from ordered probit models for mental health (Dummy for the maximum mental health level)

Explanatory Variables	Model 5	Model 6	Model 7	Model 8	Model 9
Family income	0.057(5.59)***	0.058(1.80)***	0.068 (6.33)***	0.053 (5.04)***	-
Age	-0.029 (2.34)**	-0.031(2.44)**	-0.031(2.09)***	-0.033 (2.61)***	-
Gender	-	-	-	-	0.037 (1.63)*
Asset	-	-	-	-	0.046(4.75)***
Financial stress	-0.031 (1.67)*	-0.034 (5.50)*	-	-	-
Monthly salaried	0.12 (4.14)***	-	-	-	0.094(3.41)***
Self employed	0.12 (3.34)***	-	-	-	-
Public sector	-	0.113 (2.49)**	-	-	-
Private sector	-	0.063 (2.16)**	-	-	-
Permanent job	-	-	0.030(2.65)***	-	-
Organized sector	-	-	-	0.099 (3.42)***	-
Long term disease	-0.082 (4.49)***	-0.085(4.50)***	-0.085 (4.55)***	-0.084 (4.45)***	-
Digestive disorder	-0.091 (4.41)***	-0.095 (4.51)***	-0.098 (4.60)***	-0.097 (4.59)***	-
Suicide history in family	-0.07 (3.41)***	-0.068 (3.22)***	-0.071 (3.48)***	0.072(3.58)***	-
Minority caste	-0.050 (2.60)***	-0.043 (2.19)**	-0.045 (2.23)**	-0.042 (2.06)**	-
Deaths of close one	-0.054 (2.47)***	-0.055 (2.51)***	-0.062 (2.76)***	-0.058 (2.61)***	-
Work anxiety	-0.031 (3.87)***	-0.032 (3.95)***	-0.035 (4.17)***	-0.032 (3.95)***	-
Work pressure	-0.015 (1.80)**	-	-	-	-
Political freedom	0.026 (3.33)***	0.026 (3.36)***	0.027 (3.39)***	0.025 (3.19)***	-
Safety of women	0.025 (2.73)***	0.019 (2.04)**	0.019 (2.41)**	0.019 (2.06)**	-

Table 4. (Continued).

Explanatory Variables	Model 5	Model 6	Model 7	Model 8	Model 9
Alcohol disorder	-	-	-	-	-0.062(3.02)***
Length of married life	-	-	-	-	-0.002(2.56)**
Span of emigration	-	-	-	-	-0.001 (0.79)
Number of child	-	-	-	-	
1					- 0.148 (3.69)***
2					- 0.125 (3.62)***
3+					- 0.108 (3.74)***
Leisure	-	-	-	-	-0.001 (0.19)
Social networking	-	-	-	-	0.007 (0.30)
Number of friend	-	-	-	-	0.001 (0.98)
Accrual of Wealth	-	-	-	-	-0.014 (1.71)**
Inflation	-	-	-	-	-0.022 (2.16)**
Absence of Poverty	-	-	-	-	0.022 (1.99)**
Stress-free atmosphere of Urban area	-	-	-	-	0.015 (1.94)*
Facilities of modern amenities	-	-	-	-	0.006 (0.54)
Y = Pr (mental health score = 12) =	0.120	0.123	0.124	0.122	0.136

Notes: Robust z statistics in parentheses.
*Significant at 10%; **significant at 5%; ***significant at 1%. The reported probit results are marginal effects.

The Internal consistency coefficients (Cronbach's α) have been reported for the mental health scores in Table 2. Cronbach's α tells us what proportion of the variance in the average aggregate score is accounted for by the sum of pair wise covariances and therefore not by the variances of individual dummy variables. A higher value of Cronbach's α implies that the variance in average aggregate score is driven more by the fact that the various items (questions) are measuring the same phenomenon (mental health) than phenomena specific to that highlighted by each question i.e., this score is indeed a reliable measure of mental health. The value of Cronbach's α in this case is 0.8 which tells us that the compilation of questions in the questionnaire leads to a good and reliable measure of mental health.

REFERENCES

Andrés, A.R., Chakraborty, B., Dasgupta, P. and Mitra, S. (2014). Realizing the significance of socio-economic triggers for mental health outcomes in India. *Journal of Behavioral and Experimental Economics*, 50: 50–57.

Artazcoz, L., Benach, J., Borrell, C. and Cortes, I. (2004). Unemployment and mental health, understanding the interactions among gender, family roles, and social class. *American Journal of Public Health*, 94(1): 82–88.

Avery, J., Dal Grande, E., Taylor, A. and Gill, T. (2004). Which South Australians experience psychological distress, Kessler psychological distress 10-item scale. *Adelaide, South Australia, Population Research & Outcomes Studies Unit, South Australian Department of Health.*

Ballas, D. and Dorling, D. (2007). Measuring the impact of major life events upon happiness". *International Journal of Epidemiology*, 36: 1244–1252.

Bertrand, M. and Mullainathan, S. (2001). Do people mean what they say? Implications for subjective survey data. *American Economic Review*, 91(2): 67–72.

Bohra, N., Srivastasa, S. and Bhatia, M.S. (2015). Depression in women in Indian context. *Indian Journal of Psychiatry*, 57 (Supplementary 2): S239–S245.

Bhugra, D. and Jones, P. (2001). Migration and mental illness. *Advances in Psychiatric Treatment*, 7: 216–223.

Bhugra, D. (2004). Migration and mental health. *Acta Psychiatrica Scandinavica*, 109: 243–248.

Blanchflower, D. and Oswald, A.J. (2004). Wellbeing over time in Britain and the USA. *Journal of Public Economics*, 88: 1359–1386.

Choi, B.K., Clays, E., De Bacquer, D and Karasek, R. (2008). Socioeconomic status, job strain and common mental disorders – An ecological (occupational) approach. *Scandinavian Journal of Work, Environment and Health*, Supplement 6: 22–32.

Clark, A.E. and Oswald, A.J. (1994). Unhappiness and unemployment. *The Economic Journal*, 104(424): 648–659.

Cutler, D.M. and Muney, A.L. (2006). Education and health: Evaluating theories and evidence. *NBER Working Paper* No, 12352, Cambridge, MA, 02138.

Dalgard, O. (2008). Social inequalities in mental health in Norway: Possible explanatory factors. *International Journal for Equity in Health*, 7: 27.

Das, J., Das, R.K. and Das, V. (2012). The mental health gender-gap in urban India: Patterns and narratives. *Social Science & Medicine*, 75: 1660-1672.

Das, J., Do, Q.T., Friedman, J. and McKenzie, D. (2009). Mental health patterns and consequences: results from survey data in five developing countries. *World Bank Economic Review*, 23(1): 31–55.

Das, J., Do, Q.T., Friedman, J., McKenzie, D., Scott, K. (2007). Mental health and poverty in developing countries: revisiting the relationship. *Social Science and Medicine*, 65: 467–480.

Di Tella, R., MacCulloch, R.J. and Oswald, A.J. (2001). Preferences over inflation and unemployment: Evidence from surveys of happiness. *The American Economic Review*, 91(1): 335–341.

Dube, K.C. (1970). A study of prevalence and biosocial variables in mental illness in a rural and an urban community in Uttar Pradesh. *Acta Psychiatrica Scandinavica*, 46: 327–359.

Easterlin, R.A. (1995). Will raising the incomes of all increase the happiness of all? *Journal of Economic Behavior and Organization*, 27: 35–47.

Endsley, P., Weobong, B. and Nadkarni, A. (2017). The psychometric properties of GHQ for detecting common mental disorder among community dwelling men in Goa, India. *Asian Journal of Psychiatry*, 28: 106–110.

Evenson, R.J. and Simon, R.W. (2005). Clarifying the relationship between parenthood and depression. *Journal of Health and Social Behavior*, 46: 341–358.

Firdaus, G. (2017). Mental well-being of migrants in urban center of India: Analyzing the role of social environment. *Indian Journal of Psychiatry*, 59(2): 164–169.

Frey, B.S. and Stutzer, A. (2002). What can economists learn from happiness research? *Journal of Economic Literature*, 40(2): 402–435.

Ganguli, H.C. (2000). Epidemiological finding on prevalence of mental disorders in India. *Indian Journal of Psychiatry*, 42: 14–20.

Goldsmith, A.H., Veum, J.R. and Darity, W. (1996). The impact of labor force history on self-esteem and its component parts, anxiety, alienation, and depression. *Journal of Economic Psychology*, 17(2): 183–220.

Graham, C. (2008). Happiness and health: Lessons – and questions – for public policy. *Health Affairs*, 27(1): 72–87.

Grigsby, A.B., Anderson, R.J., Freedland, K.E., Clouse, R.E. and Lustman, P.J. (2002). Prevalence of anxiety in adults with diabetes: A systematic review. *Journal of Psychosomatic Research*, 53(6): 1053–1060.

Harpham, T. (1994). Urbanization and mental health in developing countries: a research role for social scientists, public health professionals and social psychiatrists. *Social Science and Medicine*, 39 (2): 233–245.

Helliwell, J.F. (2003). How's life? Combining individual and national variables to explain subjective well-being. *Economic Modeling*, 20 (2): 331–360.

Himelhoch, S., Lehman, A., Kreyenbuhl, J., Daumit, G., Brown, C. and Dixon, L. (2004). Prevalence of chronic obstructive pulmonary disease among those with serious mental illness. *American Journal of Psychiatry*, 161 (12): 2317–2319.

Korten, A. and Henderson, S. (2000). The Australian National Survey of Mental Health and Well- Being, common psychological symptoms, and disablement. *British Journal of Psychiatry*, 177: 325–330.

Lakshmanasamy, T. (2010). Are you satisfied with your income? The economics of happiness in India. *Journal of Quantitative Economics*, 8 (2): 115–141.

Layard, R. (2005). *Happiness: Lessons from a New Science.* New York, Penguin Press.
Likert, R. (1931). *A Technique for the measurement of attitudes, Archives of Psychology*, New York, Columbia University Press.
Lincoln, K., Chatters, L. and Taylor, R. (2003). Psychological distress among black and white Americans: differential effects of social support, negative interaction, and personal control. *Journal of Health & Social Behavior*, 44: 390–407.
Nandi, D.N., Banerjee, G., Mukherjee, S.P., Sarkar, S., Boral, G.C. and Mukherjee, A. (1986). A study of psychiatric morbidity of a rural community at an interval of 10 years. *Indian Journal of Psychiatry*, 28: 179–194.
Nandi, D.N., Banerjee, G., Chowdhury, A.N., Banerjee, T., Boral, G.C. and Sen, B. (1992). Urbanisation and mental morbidity in certain tribal communities in West Bengal. *Indian Journal of Psychiatry*, 34: 334–339.
Mueser, K.T. and McGurk, S.R. (2004). *Seminar on schizophrenia. Lancet*, 363: 2063–2072.
Murthy, R.S. (1987a). Overview of psychiatric epidemiology in India. Workshop on research issues in psychiatric epidemiology in India, (unpublished). *Collaborative study on severe mental morbidity report.* Indian Council of Medical Research and Department of Science and Technology, New Delhi, 1987.
Patel, V., Araya, R., de Lima, M., Ludermir, A. and Todd, C. (1999). Women, poverty, and common mental disorders in four restructuring societies. *Social Science & Medicine*, 49: 1461–1471.
Patel, V. and Kleinman, A. (2003). Poverty and common mental disorders in developing countries. *Bulletin of the World Health Organization*, 81: 609–615.
Patel, V., Araya, R., Chowdhury, N. and King, M. (2008). Detecting common mental disorders in primary care in India: a comparison of five screening questionnaires. *Psychological Medicine*, 38(2): 221–228.

Patten, S.B. (1999). Long-term medical conditions and major depression in the Canadian population. *Canadian Journal of Psychiatry*, 44 (2):151–157.

Phillips, P. and Johnson, S. (2001). How does drug and alcohol misuse develop among people with psychotic illness? A literature review. *Social Psychiatry and Psychiatric Epidemiology*, 36(6): 269–276.

Robson, D. and Gray, R. (2007). Serious mental illness and physical health problems: A discussion paper. *International Journal of Nursing Studies*, 44: 457–466.

Raphael, B., Schmolke, M. and Wooding, S. (2005). Links between mental and physical health and illnesses. In, Herrman, H., Saxena, S., Moodie, R. (editors). Promoting mental health, concepts, emerging evidence, and practice. World Health Organization, Geneva.

Reddy, P.R., Murthy, K.K and Anand, B. (1994). An interval study of mental morbidity in a south Indian rural community in 1981–91. *Indian Journal of Social Psychiatry*, 10: 11–19.

Richardson, T., Elliott, P. and Roberts, R. (2013). The relationship between personal unsecured debt and mental and physical health: A systematic review and meta-analysis. *Clinical Psychology Review*, 33 (8): 1148–1162.

Rosenthal, L., Carroll-Scott, A., Earnshaw, V.A., Santilli, A. and Ickovics, J.R. (2012). The importance of full-time work for urban adults' mental and physical health. *Social Science & Medicine*, 75 (9): 1692–1696.

Simon, R.W. (2002). Revisiting the relationship among gender, marital status, and mental health.
The American Journal of Sociology, 107(4): 1065–1096.

Singh, S.K. and Kashyap, G.C. (2016). Mental health problems among male tannery workers: A study of Kanpur City, India. *Annals of. Psychiatry and Mental Health*, 4(7): 1089.

Singh, A. and Modi, R. (2011). Indian Ancient Thought and Well-being (Happiness). *Bilingual journal of Humanities & Social Sciences*, 2 (1 & 2): 1–4.

Srivastava, K. (2009). Urbanization and mental health. *Indian Psychiatry Journal,* 18(2): 75–76.

Stanca, L. (2012). Suffer the little children: Measuring the effects of parenthood on well-being world-wide. *Journal of Economic Behavior and Organization*, 81: 742–750.

Tannenbaum, C.J., Lexchin, Tamblyn, R. and Romans, S. (2009). Indicators for measuring mental health: Towards better surveillance. *Health Policy*, 5(2): 177–186.

The Centre for Genetics Education (2012). *Mental illness and inherited predisposition- schizophrenia and bipolar disorder.* www.genetics.edu.au/genetics/Genetic-conditions-supportgroups/FS58KBS.pdf [accessed 8th September 2017].

Umberson, D. (1993). Socio-demographic position, world views, and psychological distress. *Social Science Quarterly*,74: 575–589.

Whelan, C.T. (1992). The role of income, life-style deprivation, and financial strain in mediating the impact of unemployment on psychological distress: Evidence from the Republic of Ireland. *Journal of Occupational and Organisational Psychology*, 65: 331–344.

Wheaton, B. (1990). Life transitions, role histories, and mental health. *American Sociological Review*, 55 (2): 209–223.

World Health Organization (2017). Depression in India. Let's talk. http://www.searo.who.int/india/depression_in_india.pdf [accessed 18th March 2018]

Veenhoven, R. (2000). Freedom and happiness: A comparative study in forty-four nations in the early 1990's in Culture and Subjective Well-Being. Ed Diener and Eunkook M. Suh, eds. in *Culture and Subjective Wellbeing*. Cambridge, MA, MIT Press, 257–288.

Verghese, A., Beig, A., Senseman, L.A., Rao, S.S. and Benjamin, V. (1973). A social and psychiatric study of a representative group of families in Vellore town. *Indian Journal Medical Research*, 61: 608–620.

Vijayakumar, L. (2007). Suicide and its prevention, the urgent need in India. *Indian Journal of Psychiatry*, 49: 81–84.

In: A Socio-Economic and Demographic ... ISBN: 978-1-53619-023-6
Editors: A. Rodriguez Andres et al. © 2021 Nova Science Publishers, Inc.

Chapter 2

SUICIDE IN INDIA

David Lester[1,], Bijou Yang[2] and Kavita Naik[3]*

[1]Stockton University, NJ, US
[2]Drexel University, PA, US
[3]The Richard Stockton College of New Jersey, NJ, US

ABSTRACT

The Indian suicide rate has been rising in recent years, from 6.3 per 100,000 per year in 1980 to 10.9 in 2009, 10.6 in 2015 and 10.4 in 2019, and the suicide rate varies greatly over the regions of India, ranging from 0.0 in Lakshadweep to 33.1 in Sikkim in 2019. The present study was designed to investigate whether socioeconomic indicators were associated with the time-series and regional variation in suicide rates in India. Over time, urbanization and life expectancy were associated with the suicide rate (positively and negatively, respectively). Over the regions, the proportion of Muslims, the proportion of children and the relative proportion of male children were each negatively associated with the

---

[*] Corresponding Author's E-mail: david.lester@stockton.edu.

suicide rate. Limitations in the consistent and reliable collection of data in India impair better studies of the suicide rate in India.

Keywords: suicide rates, India, time series

INTRODUCTION

Suicide is a growing public health problem in India. The suicide rate rose from 6.3 per 100,000 per year in 1978 to 8.9 in 1990 (Radhakrishnan and Andrade, 2012), and the suicide rate has risen very year since 2001 (Srivastava, 2013). In 2019, the suicide rate was 10.4. According to WHO data[3], the crude suicide rates in India in 2015 were 17.1 for men and 14.1 for women. Suicide ranks in the top ten leading causes of death of adults and in the top three leading causes of death for young adults (aged 16-35 years) (Salve et al., 2013). The suicide rate also varies greatly over the Indian states, ranging from 0.0 in Lakshadweep to 33.1 in Sikkim in 2019.

THEORIES OF SUICIDE

In the 19th Century, Emile Durkheim (1897) argued that variables at the societal (aggregate) level, especially socioeconomic variables, were important determinants of suicide rates. Durkheim proposed two abstract constructs, social integration, and social regulation, in order to explain the regional and temporal variation in suicide rates. Social integration is the degree to which the members of a society are bound together in social relationships, while social regulation is the degree to which people's desires and behavior are constrained by social norms and rules. Durkheim proposed that moderate levels of social integration and social regulation result in a lower suicide rate. Low levels of social integration and social regulation result in high rates of egoistic suicide and anomic suicide,

---

[3] http://apps.who.int/gho/data/node.main.MHSUICIDE?lang = en.

respectively, whereas high levels of social integration and social regulation result in high rates of altruistic suicide and fatalistic suicide, respectively. Later theorists, however, have argued that altruistic and fatalist suicides are rare in modern societies, and so Durkheim's theory of suicide can be restated as low levels of social integration and regulation resulting in high rates of suicide (Johnson, 1965).

Developed nations have excellent government data collection agencies which produce regional and time-series data for many socioeconomic indicators. Lester and Yang (1998) examined predictors of national suicide rates over time for 36 nations for the period 1950-1985 and found, for example, that divorce rates were a much more consistent predictor of suicide rates than were marriage rates. Lester (1998-1999) reviewed studies of the regional variation in suicide rates within 14 nations and found that residential stability and migration were the strongest correlates of regional suicide rates within a nation, negatively and positively, respectively. These data support Durkheim's theory of suicide as modified by Johnson.

Economic variables can also be incorporated into this theory of suicide. Lester and Yang (1997) noted that, according to Durkheim's theory, when the economy expands or contracts sharply, both social integration and social regulation may weaken, thereby resulting in a higher suicide rate. This produces a U-shaped function. However, Yang and Lester noted that there are two competing theories: (i) Ginsberg's procyclical theory (suicide rates are higher during economic expansions), and (ii) Henry and Short's countercyclical theory (suicide rates are higher during economic recessions).

Ginsberg (1966) argued that suicide arose from the dissatisfaction of individuals. Dissatisfaction itself was related directly to the discrepancy between the actual reward that individuals were receiving and their level of aspiration. Ginsberg assumed that the actual reward varies positively with the business cycle. When replacing the individual level of dissatisfaction, reward, and aspiration with the average levels for the society, suicidal behavior at the societal level may be seen as resulting from the discrepancy between aspirations and rewards. As the economy expands toward the peak of the business cycle, the prosperous economic environment pushes aspirations up at a rate faster than the rewards. The resulting growing disparity between aspirations and rewards triggers suicide. When the economy faces a recession, as it moves toward the trough of the business cycle, aspirations drop faster than rewards, thus shrinking the disparity between aspirations and rewards. As a result, the suicide rate will decline.

Henry and Short (1954) argued that the relationship between suicide and business cycle is countercyclical. Suicide rates tend to rise during times of economic busts and to fall during times of economic booms. Their theory is based on a frustration-aggression hypothesis which is grounded in five assumptions: (a) frustration often results in aggression; (b) business cycles affect the hierarchical rankings of persons by status; (c) frustrations are caused by a failure to maintain a constant or rising position in the status hierarchy relative to the status position of other groups; (d) high-status persons lose status relative to low status persons during business contractions, and they gain relative status during business expansions; and (e) suicide occurs mainly in high-status persons. During business contractions, some individuals of high economic status commit suicide due to their loss of status relative to low-status individuals, whereas during expansions, individuals of high status tend to gain relative status and so are less inclined to kill themselves.

As Lester (Lester, B., 2001) has pointed out, all these theories imply a mediational model by which economic cycles affect suicide rates. In Durkheim's theory, the mediating variables are social integration and social regulation, in Ginsberg's theory, the mediating variable is aspiration level relative to actual rewards received and, in Henry and Short's theory, the mediating factor is the relative status of social groups.

Innamorati et al. (2017) reviewed research on the impact of the economy on suicide and concluded that there was no consistent evidence that economic recessions or economic expansions result in higher suicide rates. Some studies report a deleterious impact on suicide rates from recessions, some report a deleterious impact from expansions, while others report mixed impacts or no impact at all. It appears that the association varies greatly by country and, also by the sex, age and employment status of the population group studied.

SUICIDE IN INDIA

For India, data for socioeconomic indicators over time and over the different regions are not as detailed and not as consistently available. Therefore, it has been difficult to conduct time-series and ecological studies of the variation in the suicide rate. Lester and Naik (2015) explored whether social indicators could be identified that correlate with the Indian suicide rate over time and over the states of India.

TIME SERIES

Lester and Naik (2015) studied the time period from 1967 to 2009. The total suicide rate is shown in Table 1 and Figure 1, and the suicide rates by sex are shown in Table 1. Although the suicide rate declined from 1970 to 1980, overall there was a general increase over the 43-year period (Pearson $r = 0.79$), and the same was true for the male and female suicide rates for the period 1973-2009 ($r = 0.93$ and 0.84, respectively). The male/female suicide rate ratio also increased over this time period ($r = 0.54$), indicating that the male suicide rate increased at a higher rate than the female suicide rate. The period of most rapid growth in the suicide rate was in the 1980s, and the rate appears to have stabilized in the 21st century.

It was possible to calculate suicide rates by the major methods for suicide (see Table 1).

Over the 43-year period from 1967 to 2009, the suicide rates by fire, hanging and poisons increased ($r = 0.85$, 0.95 and 0.89, respectively), while the suicide rates by drowning and guns decreased ($r = -0.87$ and -0.42, respectively).

Table 1. Suicide rates in India, 1967-2009

year	total	male	female	m/f/	drown	fire	gun	hang	poison	ratio
1967	7.7	-	-	-	1.9	0.4	0.08	1.4	1.3	
1968	8.0	-	-	-	1.9	0.4	0.07	1.5	1.6	
1969	8.4	-	-	-	1.8	0.5	0.07	1.5	1.8	
1970	9.1	-	-	-	1.8	0.5	0.10	1.5	2.2	
1971	7.9	-	-	-	1.4	0.4	0.07	1.5	2.2	
1972	7.7	-	-	-	1.4	0.5	0.06	1.4	2.3	
1973	7.1	8.5	5.7	1.51	1.3	0.4	0.05	1.3	2.1	
1974	7.8	9.2	6.5	1.42	1.3	0.5	0.06	1.4	2.2	
1975	7.1	8.5	5.9	1.44	1.1	0.4	0.07	1.4	2.1	
1976	6.8	7.7	5.9	1.29	1.3	0.5	0.09	1.3	2.0	
1977	6.3	7.3	5.4	1.34	1.2	0.4	0.04	1.3	1.8	
1978	6.3	7.4	5.3	1.42	1.2	0.4	0.06	1.3	1.5	
1979	5.9	6.9	4.9	1.41	1.2	0.4	0.06	1.3	1.3	
1980	6.3	7.2	5.5	1.29	1.1	0.5	0.08	1.5	1.5	
1981	5.8	6.9	5.1	1.36	1.0	0.5	0.08	1.4	1.3	
1982	6.5	7.5	5.5	1.36	1.0	0.5	0.05	1.6	1.7	
1983	6.4	7.5	5.7	1.32	0.9	0.6	0.05	1.6	1.7	
1984	6.8	7.9	6.1	1.28	1.0	0.6	0.05	1.6	2.1	
1985	7.0	8.0	6.3	1.27	0.9	0.7	0.06	1.7	2.1	
1986	7.1	8.0	6.4	1.26	0.9	0.7	0.06	1.7	2.2	
1987	7.5	8.6	6.6	1.31	0.9	0.7	0.06	1.9	2.3	
1988	8.1	9.3	7.0	1.32	1.0	0.7	0.07	2.0	2.5	
1989	8.5	9.6	7.4	1.31	1.0	0.8	0.07	2.1	2.8	
1990	8.9	10.2	7.7	1.32	1.0	0.8	0.06	2.2	3.0	
1991	9.2	10.6	8.0	1.34	1.1	0.9	0.07	2.1	3.0	
1992	9.2	10.7	7.9	1.35	0.9	0.8	0.06	2.2	3.2	
1993	9.5	11.0	8.2	1.35	1.0	1.1	0.08	2.3	3.3	
1994	9.9	11.4	8.4	1.34	0.9	1.1	0.07	2.3	3.4	
1995	9.7	11.0	8.4	1.32	1.0	1.1	0.07	2.4	3.7	
1996	9.5	10.6	8.2	1.29	0.9	1.1	0.04	2.5	3.5	
1997	10.0	11.4	8.6	1.32	0.9	1.1	0.07	2.7	3.7	
1998	10.8	12.3	9.2	1.34	1.0	1.2	0.09	2.8	4.0	
1999	11.2	12.8	9.4	1.35	1.0	1.2	0.06	2.8	4.2	
2000	10.8	12.6	8.7	1.45	0.9	1.2	0.05	2.8	4.1	
2001	10.6	12.5	8.7	1.44	0.8	1.1	0.04	2.9	4.1	
2002	10.5	12.8	8.1	1.58	0.8	1.0	0.04	3.0	3.9	
2003	10.4	12.8	7.9	1.62	0.7	1.0	0.05	3.1	4.0	
2004	10.5	13.0	7.8	1.66	0.7	0.8	0.05	3.3	3.9	
2005	10.3	12.8	7.7	1.67	0.7	0.8	0.07	3.3	3.8	
2006	10.5	13.1	7.8	1.67	0.8	0.9	0.03	3.4	3.7	
2007	10.8	13.5	7.9	1.72	0.7	0.9	0.06	3.4	3.8	
2008	10.8	13.5	7.9	1.70	0.7	0.9	0.04	3.5	3.8	
2009	10.9	12.7	9.3	1.37	0.7	1.0	0.05	3.4	3.7	

Life expectancy and the urban population percentage increased over the 43-year period (r = 0.99 and 0.998, respectively), GDP growth also increased over the period (r = 0.39), although less steadily, while the birth rate declined (r = -0.99). The suicide rate was positively associated with all the social indicators over this period: 0.36 with GDP growth, 0.69 with life expectancy, 0.75 with the percentage of the urban population, and -0.86 with the birth rate. However, since all of these variables had a linear association with time, these positive correlations are probably simply a result of the linear trends. In a multiple regression (see Table 2), the time series suicide rate was predicted by the percentage of the population that is urban (positively) and life expectancy (negatively).

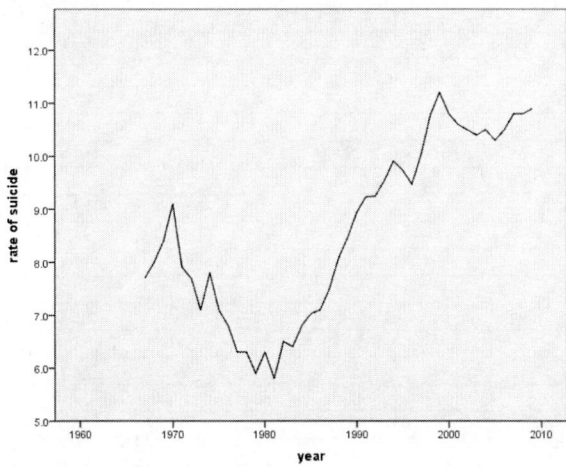

Figure 1. The total Indian suicide rate by year, 1967-2009.

Table 2. Predicting the time-series suicide rate using multiple regressions (beta coefficients shown)

	Suicide Rate			
	Total	Male	Female	Male/Female ratio
% urban population	4.75***#	4.12***#	2.45#	5.38*#
GDP growth	-0.04	-0.01	-0.02	0.00
life expectancy	-4.01***#	-3.21***#	-1.63	-4.86*#
R^2	0.79	0.86	0.68	0.38

* p < .05
** p < .01
*** P < .001
# Significant in the backward multiple regression.

REGIONAL STUDY OVER THE INDIAN STATES

Table 3. Suicide rates of the regions of India in 2010 and 2019 (From the National Crime Records Bureau, India)

States	2010	2019
Andhra Pradesh[4]	18.9	12.4
Arunchal Pradesh	10.6	7.4
Assam	9.7	6.9
Bihar	1.3	0.5
Chhattisgarh	26.6	26.4
Goa	18.5	16.8
Gujurat	10.7	11.2
Haryana	11.8	14.5
Himachal Pradesh	8.1	8.0
Jammu & Kashmir	1.9	2.1
Jharkhand	4.0	4.4
Karnataka	21.5	16.1
Kerala	24.6	24,3
Madhya Pradesh	12.5	15.1
Manipur	1.4	1.0
Maharashtra	14.5	15.4
Meghalay	4.1	6.1
Mizoram	7.5	5.9
Nagaland	0.5	1.9
Orissa	10.4	10.5
Punjab	3.4	7.9
Rajasthan	7.3	5.2
Sikkim	45.9	33.1
Tamil Nadu	24.5	17.8
Telangana	20.6	
Tripura	20.1	18.2
Uttar Pradesh	1.8	2.4
Uttarkhand	2.9	4.6
West Bengal	17.8	13.0
Union Territories		
Andaman & Nicobar Islands	36.1	45.5
Chandigarh	6.3	11.1
Dadra & Nagar Haveli	22.3	17.1
Delhi (UT)	8.4	12.7
Daman & Diu	15.5	10.9
Laskhadweep	1.4	0.0
Pondicherry	45.5	32.5

---

[4] Recently, in 2014, Telangana was established as a state independent of Andhra Pradesh.

The suicide rate varied considerably over the states and union territories of India, ranging from 0.5 per 100,000 per year in Nagaland in 2010 to 45.9 in Sikkim (see Table 3). Lester and Naik (2015) focused on the year 2010. The correlations between the social indicators and the suicide rates of the regions are shown in Table 4. At the bivariate level, only the presence of children predicted the regional suicide rate. Regions with a greater proportion of male children (versus female children) and with a higher proportion of children in the population had lower suicide rates. However, in the multiple regression, two additional predictors of regional suicide rates were identified. The regions with a higher proportion of Muslims had lower suicide rates, and the Indian *states* had lower suicide rates than the Indian *union territories*.

Table 4. Correlations of the social indicators with suicide rates over the 35 regions of India

2010 Suicide rate and	Correlation (Pearson r)	Multiple Regression (beta)
Population growth	-0.02	0.18
m/f children	-0.42*	-0.28#
% children	-0.39*	-0.50*#
% Muslim	-0.27	-0.32#
Pop den	-0.07	-0.27
Rural	-0.05	0.14
Literacy	0.29	-0.06
m/f adults	-0.03	-0.28
population	-0.16	0.12
state(1) vs.territories(0)	-0.24	-0.64*#
Multiple R	0.73	

* p < .05
\# significant in a backward multiple regression.

DISCUSSION

The time series analysis of the Indian suicide rate indicated that the suicide rate was positively associated with the proportion of the urban population but negatively associated with the life expectancy. An earlier analysis for the period 1969-1988 was able to study different social indicators and found that the time-series Indian suicide rate was predicted by the participation of women in the labor force (positively) and by fertility (negatively) (Lester et al., 1999).

The only correlates of the regional suicide rates identified were the percentage of children and the relative predominance of male children. In previous research, Pandey (1986) found that the regional suicide rates were associated with population density, as did Lester et al. (1999), while the present analysis no longer found this association using data from 2010. Lester (1996) found that the regional suicide rates were not associated with the percentages of Muslims in each region, but the present analysis found a weak negative association in the multiple regression analysis. These results indicate the importance of replicating older findings with more recent data since socioeconomic development may change the pattern of associations.

Fertility rates were not available for the union territories but were available for the states. For the 28 states in 2010, the association between suicide rates and fertility rates was negative ($r = -0.60$, $p = .001$). The higher the fertility rate, the lower the suicide rate.

A major limitation of this study, along with previous research on suicide in India is the unreliability of official data on suicide from India. Rane and Nadkarni (2014) identified 36 studies on suicide in India and found that suicide rates based on examination of local medical examiner records often reported higher suicide rates than the official suicide rates, with rates as high as 95 per 100,000 per year in some villages as compared to an official suicide rate of 11. Rane and Nadkarni concluded that the quality of information about suicide was "quite limited" (p. 69). Suicide is illegal in India, as it is in many other nations, including Ghana and Singapore (Kahn and Lester, 2013). The illegality of suicide increases the likelihood that suicidal deaths will be covered up and misclassified (typically as accidental). In a study of seven nations that decriminalized suicide, Lester (2002) found that the official suicide rate after decriminalization was higher than in the years prior to decriminalization. If and when the Indian courts decriminalize suicide, more accurate mortality rates may be possible.

Another major limitation is the paucity of consistent information over time and over the regions of India for important socioeconomic variables. Research into the ecological and time-series variation in the Indian suicide rates would be greatly facilitated were a reliable and complete data sets for these variables made available. However, it is hoped that this preliminary study will stimulate further research on suicide in India.

REFERENCES

Durkheim E. (1897). *Le Suicide*. Paris, France: Felix Alcan.
Ginsberg, R.B. (1966). Anomie and aspirations. *Dissertation Abstracts*, 27A: 3945–3946.
Henry, A.F. and Short, J.F. (1954). *Suicide and Homicide*. New York: Free Press.
Innamorati, M., Pompili, M., Lester, D. and Yang, B. (2017). Economic crises and suicide. In O. Wilson-Flores (Ed.) *Economic Crises*, pp. 123-138. Hauppauge, NY: Nova.
Kahn, D.L. and Lester, D. (2013). Efforts to decriminalize suicide in Ghana, India and Singapore. *Suicidology Online*, 4: 110–118.
Lester, B.Y. (2001). Learnings from Durkheim and beyond: the economy and suicide. *Suicide & Life-Threatening Behavior*, 31: 15–31.
Lester, D. (1996). Suicide in Indian states and religion. *Psychological Reports*, 79: 342.
Lester, D. (1998,1999). Correlates of regional suicide rates. *Omega*, 38: 99–102.
Lester, D. (2002). Decriminalization of suicide in seven nations and suicide rates. *Psychological Reports*, 91: 898.
Lester, D. and Naik, K. (2015). Suicide in India. *Current Politics & Economics of Northern & Western Asia*, 24(4): 543–551.
Lester, D. and Yang B.J. (1997). *The Economy and Suicide: Economic Perspectives on Suicide*. Commack, NY: Nova Science.
Lester, D. and Yang, B.J. (1998). *Suicide and Homicide in the 20th Century*. Commack, NY: Nova Science.

Pandey, R. (1986). Suicide and social structure in India. *Social Defense*, 21(83): 5–29.

Radhakrishnan, R. and Andrade, C. (2012). Suicide: an Indian perspective. *Indian Journal of Psychiatry*, 54: 304–319.

Rane, A. and Nadkarni, A. (2014). Suicide in India: a systematic review. *Shanghai Archives of Psychiatry*, 26(2): 69–80.

Salve, H., Kumar, R., Sinha, S. and Krishnan, A. (2013). Suicide and emerging public health problem. *Indian Journal of Public Health*, 57: 40–42.

Srivastava, A. (2013). Psychological attributes and socio-demographic profile of hundred completed suicide victims in the state of Goa, India. *Indian Journal of Psychiatry*, 55: 268–272.

United Nations. (Annual). *Demographic Yearbook*. New York: United Nations.

In: A Socio-Economic and Demographic ...   ISBN: 978-1-53619-023-6
Editors: A. Rodriguez Andres et al.   © 2021 Nova Science Publishers, Inc.

Chapter 3

WHAT LEADS TO HAPPINESS AMONG CHRONICALLY ILL INDIVIDUALS?

Debangana Chakraborty[1,*] *and Anindita Chaudhuri*[2]
[1]Department of Psychology, South Calcutta Girls' College,
Kolkata, India
[2]Department of Psychology, University of Calcutta,
Kolkata, India

ABSTRACT

Chronic illnesses, for obvious reasons, can affect happiness adversely. Yet it has been observed that people with the same type of chronic illness and similar circumstances exhibit varying levels of happiness. A hypothesis is that there is a lot of variation in, the way people view the world i.e., the extent to which they adopt coping mechanisms, the nature of coping mechanisms adopted and their emotional intelligence (the ability to regulate one's own emotions, read the emotions of others and then respond positively). Note that these

---

[*] Corresponding Author's E-mail: anicaluniv@gmail.com.

factors are in turn an outcome of the interaction of nature and nurture. Through an in-depth literature review and a primary survey, the authors establish that this hypothesis is indeed true.

Keywords: happiness, emotions, chronic illnesses

INTRODUCTION

The concept of happiness came into the limelight with the emergence of the field of positive psychology in the twenty first century. Until then the focus of modern psychology was on negativity. Seligman and Csikzenthmehyle (2000) note, 'modern psychology focused too much and too long on the negative side of the polarity on anxiety, anger, depression etc., and it is time to shift our focus on happiness, joy, contentment, and so on'. So, it is evident that positive psychology emphasizes the necessity to move away from 'searching negativity and curing it' to 'searching positivity and nurturing it' for a better life. This field focuses on how people can live better by enhancing their strengths and positive qualities. It focuses on positive traits, positive emotions and, positive relationships and assumes that identifying and enhancing these can lead to a positive growth and development in human beings. Happiness and wellbeing are core and very important themes of positive psychology. As Seligman says positive psychology is all about happiness. In fact, the role of positive psychology at the subjective level is characterized by the concept of flow, optimism, hope and, well-being along with happiness.

A LOOK INTO HAPPINESS

Extensive research has been carried out in the past decade on happiness. Some researchers have explored the path to reach it and others have explored its advantages in human life. Though happiness has come into focus very recently in the field of psychology it is not a new concept in Indian culture. In ancient India, happiness literature was a much celebrated concept. The ultimate aim or manifestation of a human life was considered to be happiness. The Vedas, the Upanishada, the Bhagavad Gita, the CharakaSamhita give us the light to see happiness from the ancient Indian perspective. Advaita Vedanta a subschool of Vedanta used the term 'jiva' for 'person' (Paranjpe and Rao, 2008). Advaita Vedanta conceptualised 'jiva' as made up of five layers. The outermost layer is called 'annamayakosa' or 'sustained by food'; the second layer is called ' pranamayakosa' or 'layer of the vital breath'; the third layer is 'manmayakosa' or 'mental layer'; the fourth layer is vijyanmayakosa' or 'cognitive layer' and the innermost layer is 'anandamayakosa' or 'the joyous layer'. This layer is described as joyous because it reflects bliss (anandapratibimba) which is the characteristic of Atman or true self and identical with the Brahman, the ultimate reality. In this ultimate stage the experience of bliss and the experiencer is no longer separate (Singh, 2015).

Indian thinkers have distinguished between the concepts of 'Ananda' (happiness) from the concept of 'Sukha' (pleasure). For them 'Ananda' is a more sustainable sense of well-being and 'Sukha' is conditioned by spatio-temporal limitations of life (Salagame, 2015) that means 'Sukha' is material dependent, and materials are not finite, it is limited and impermanent. This 'Ananda' can be conceptualised as the Greek concept of 'eudaimonia'. Psychologists who believe that there has to be meaning with happiness, accept the concept of 'eudaimonia'. If a person has a purpose in life, is moving forward towards fulfilling potential in a pursuit - it has a good human life characterised by eudaimonia or happiness. Meaning lies not in pursuit of happiness, but in happiness of pursuit (Franklin, 2010). Fulfilling one's potential, whatever it is, gives sense of purpose or meaning with happiness. According to them, hedonic pleasure alone cannot bring sustainable happiness. This is well illustrated by Prince Gautama leaving the hedonic pleasures of a royal life, to search for happiness, and became Buddha, the enlightened person. Buddha was born as Siddhartha in the Sakyan clan. Siddhartha was born as a prince in Lumbini, near Kapilabastu, now Nepal. He lived during 5th century B.C. He observed that human life is full of sufferings and sorrow. He was deeply moved by the sufferings of human. He realised only spiritual enlightenment can give 'moksha' or 'nirvana' from the sufferings of life. He left his dynasty, wife, and son to search for spiritual enlightenment.

Theories of happiness conceptualised happiness from three different perspectives (Snyder et al., 2011). First, need/goal satisfaction theory says that when a goal is reached it reduces tension and yields a satisfaction of need which leads to happiness. Second, the genetic and personality predisposition theory tends to see it as stable. These researchers believe that there is a set point for happiness, a general level of happiness, which is stable in a person. Life changes may lower or raise the level of happiness but again it comes back to a stable level after proper adaptation with change. The third theory is process or activity theory, which gives the concept of 'flow'. Csikszentmihayi's concept of flow sheds light on 'happiness of pursuit' and not 'pursuit of happiness'. Csikszentmihayi and his colleagues (Csikszentmihayi et al., 1993) worked with teenagers possessed with some or the other kind of talent and found that they enjoyed pursuing their interests. The simple joy of pursuing their interest area was an intrinsic motivation which contributed to the development of these youths and contributed to their happiness. Csikszentmihayi called this intrinsic motivation 'flow'. In 'flow' people become engrossed in what they are doing. Through experience of the effect of sustaining the activity and creating pleasure it develops the mind. When a person is expected to perform in a task, the capability of the person needs to match the demand of that task. Only if the demand of the task matches the capability of the person to carry on the task then the person will have complete control over the situation. Thus, confidence grows in the person to successfully accomplish the task. The sense of self then gets replaced by a feeling of 'exhilaration'. Csikszentmihayi called this optimum experience 'flow'.

Veenhoven (1997) viewed happiness differently. For him the extent of happiness can be gauged from an overall evaluation of life. Marinic and Brkljacic (2008) said in a similar vein. "Happiness is a positive emotion or feeling of satisfaction". Thus, it depends on the degree to which a person evaluates his or her life to be positive. According to this school of thought a person determines whether the life he or she is living is worthwhile, and this determination comes from within with no external or objective evaluation being superior to this subjective evaluation of life for happiness (Diener 2000). As this evaluation is subjective, even Veenhoven (1997) could not determine the criteria a person will use for self-evaluation.

Conceptual Referent Theory by Rojas (2005) shares the same opinion. It suggests that people may define 'happiness' and the concept of a 'happy life' differently because of difference in their social and cultural backgrounds as well as nurture. Moreover, happiness and the factors that lead to it may not be equally important for everybody. How a person will look for happiness will be determined by the genetic predisposition as well as environmental factors. Thus, a negative situation or an event might not always lead to a mental breakdown in a person as the same negative event might be viewed by different people differently with some triumphing over it to lead a happy life.

CHRONIC ILLNESS AND HAPPINESS

We now look at the relationship between chronic illness and happiness as well as the relationship among chronic illness, happiness, and coping. Sometimes in life negative events can become life changing experiences or turning points (Clausen; 1993; Wethington, 2003). Accomplishments or success are not only the determining factors for growth or strength, sufferings may also serve as contributory factors for development. Health problems can be major turning points (Wethington, 2003). A new line of research unfolds the impact of happiness on health. Some studies found that happiness has strengthened the immune system (Kamen-Siegel et al., 1991; Segertrom, et al., 1998). Koopsman et al. (2010) found happiness as predicting lower mortality, which may partly be mediated by more physical activity and lower morbidity.

The nature of chronic illness allows it to develop gradually and be integrated with life. The patients are expected to accept lifestyle changes and adhere to treatment procedures. Note that, chronic illness is a potential threat to the wellbeing of individuals, as people have to live with it for a large portion of their lives. How people can live a happy life in spite of illness is a relevant question today. Chronic illness has become a national concern in the Indian context because of its interference with different aspects of life and the resulting loss in productivity and national income apart from an exacerbating effect on mortality. The cumulative loss in national income is expected to be doubled by 2030 (WHO, 2005). Cardiovascular disorder, diabetes mellitus, chronic obstructive pulmonary disease (COPD) and cancer are expected to increase in prevalence in the near future (Taylor, 2010).

If chronic illness is such a strong threat to human life, then, wellbeing and happiness of people suffering from it must be in danger. The English philosopher Jeremy Bentham notes, 'the common end of every person's effort is happiness'. If it is so, then how individuals with chronic illness manage to be happy is worth exploring. Researchers are investigating the relationship between chronic illness and happiness. If we trace back the journey of this investigation, we can see that in 1980's common pillars of enquiry were suffering (Charmaz, 1983), loss (Duval, 1984), sick role (Stewart and Sullivan, 1982) etc. The focus for a long time was on illness, deficiency, and impairment (Meyers, 2000). Emphasis was given on negative consequences of living with chronic illness. But Thorne and Peterson in 1998 questioned whether it is right to view chronic illness as just devastating or whether it should be seen as an experience which includes both joy and sorrow. Soon the focus shifted to themes such as courage and hope, reshaping of self; regaining of control, meaningfulness, etc. (Thorne and Peterson, 1998). It was seen that people with disability experienced happiness from the ability to deal with their condition (Albrecht and Devlieger, 1999; Marinic and Brjljacic, 2008). Hoppe (2013) described chronic illness as a source of happiness. The author found a paradoxical relationship between chronic illness and happiness, two seemingly mutual exclusive states. After talking to people suffering from multiple sclerosis it was concluded that people can be happy in spite of suffering from illness. Moreover, happiness could be a consequence of the suffering.

Overall, this shift to see chronic illness from a positivist view and exploring the concept of happiness within life of chronic illness sufferers brought the concept of coping and positive emotion in light, with most researches emphasizing on the role of the ability to deal with chronic illness and presence of positive emotional experiences in stimulating happiness.

CHRONIC ILLNESS, HAPPINESS, AND COPING

Relatively few studies have explored the coping strategies among chronically ill patient groups. If patients of chronic illness have to adjust successfully with the disease that they must somehow integrate their illness into their lives because all chronic illnesses require some alteration in activities and management. Hence coping is essential factor in a chronically ill patient's adjustment. How a patient appraises the chronic illness, for example, as threatening or challenging, leads to the initiation of coping efforts. Lazarus (1974) referred to coping as problem solving efforts made by an individual when the demands that he/she faces are highly relevant to his welfare and when these demands tax his adaptive resources. There are different kinds of coping. *Problem focussed coping* constitutes efforts aimed primarily at directly changing or managing a threatening or harmful stressor. *Emotion focussed coping* constitutes efforts to regulate the emotional impact of a stressful situation or provide relief from it. In this context *social support* refers to the resources provided by other people.

In general, the use of active, problem focussed strategies have been associated with positive outcomes among patients with chronic illness (e.g., Newman et al., 1990) and seeking information (Felton and Revenson, 1984) has been associated with less emotional distress. Perhaps the key to good coping is flexibility, i.e., the ability to adapt one's coping to the demands of the situation. What is clear is that no one form of coping will be effective in dealing with all stressors and the use of knowledge and wisdom to determine the extent of reliance on different forms of coping is important.

Some researchers have linked the selection of coping mechanism to genetic factors. Task oriented, emotion oriented and avoidance oriented coping styles were pointed as moderately heritable, although their phenotypic (observable overt expression of the coping styles which are result of interaction of genetic factors with environmental factors) variance were contributed by considerable environmental factors (Navrady et al., 2018). Early life experiences were also given importance as building blocks of coping behaviour (Langenhof and Komedur, 2018). The influence of environmental factors, such as family background, on coping behaviour is well accepted. On the other hand, personality is also seen as being determined by genetic factors. Hence the role of heredity in coping behaviour cannot be denied. Therefore, how a person copes with chronic illness varies across persons. Naturally whether a patient with chronic illness will live with it happily or report negative effects and lowered wellbeing depends on coping styles selected by him/her.

Some studies have explored the relationship between coping and happiness. An Indian study found that social support contributed positively to happiness of female youths (Saha et al., 2015). This finding is supported by another study by Chan and Lee (2006): a study of 2000 Chinese elderly people revealed that a larger social support network resulted in greater happiness among the elderly. This relationship between happiness and social support did not change with social and demographic factors. Babamiri et al's (2014) exploration of chronic illness patients assessed 100 hospitalised cardiovascular patients and found that task oriented coping was the best predictor of happiness along with negative automatic thought and life quality.

Chronic Illness, Happiness, and Emotional Intelligence

The term *Emotional Intelligence* was coined by Salovey and Mayer and popularized by Daniel Goleman. As soon as emotional intelligence started to grab interest of researchers, it was equated with everything from 'zeal and persistence' (Goleman, 1995) to 'general character' (Gowing, 2001). Bar-On defined EI as a composite of different facets comprising cognitive, motivational, and affective constructs. Mowrer (1960) suggested that emotion was "a high order of intelligence". In the same way Salovey and Mayer (1990) theorized that cognitive abilities and emotional skills are essential for adapting behaviour properly to circumstances. Salovey and Mayer (1990) proposed a formal definition of emotional intelligence as "The ability to monitor one's own and others' feelings, to discriminate among them, and to use this information to guide one's thinking and action." A study by Brackett and Mayer (2003) reveals the same result. EI was found to be highly correlated with happiness with a domain overlap of about 60%. It reflects that some of the influencing factors of happiness and emotional intelligence are similar. Furnham and Petrides (2008) also found positive association between EI and happiness, thus supporting Bar-On's finding. It is shown by the literatures that people with high emotional intelligence are on an average more successful in managing and solving emotional problems, and hence manage stress well and maintain positive and productive family and social lives (Mathews and Zeidner, 2000). As emotional intelligence helps to manage emotions and interpersonal relationships well (Lopes, et al. 2004), it decreases negative emotions and increases positive affects. People who experience positive affects frequently are those that have a tendency for experiencing positive emotions frequently and interacting with others and life's changes in a positive way, and thus tend to have higher happiness (Lyubomirsky et al., 2005).

Some other studies have found a positive relationship between happiness and emotional intelligence. Pahuja et al. (2016) found a strong relationship between emotional intelligence and happiness while exploring the roles of occupational stress and emotional intelligence as exogenous determinants of individual happiness for employees of manufacturing and service sectors in India. They concluded that management of occupational stress through emotional intelligence has direct and indirect effects on individual happiness. A 12-week follow up study by Ruiz-Aranda et al. (2014) examined the relationship between emotional intelligence and well-being indicators (life satisfaction and happiness). 264 female nursing students completed tasks for the evaluation of an ability measure of emotional intelligence. After 12 weeks, participants were administered questionnaires to evaluate the Perceived Stress Scale, Satisfaction with Life Scale and Subjective Happiness Scale. Participants with higher EI reported less perceived stress and higher levels of life satisfaction and happiness. The results of this study suggest that perceived stress mediates the relationship between EI and well-being indicators, specifically life satisfaction and happiness. A study by Ara (2013) also tried to find out the relationship between emotional intelligence and happiness. Results revealed significant gender difference in emotional intelligence with females scoring higher. Emotional intelligence was found to be significantly correlated with happiness. Sasanpour et al. (2012) conducted a study of 120 students of medical science to find out whether emotional intelligence is related to happiness and mental health. The three tools used in this study were 1) Bar-On Emotional Intelligence Questionnaire, 2) Goldberg and Williams's Mental Health Questionnaire (GHQ), and 3) Argyl and Lou's Oxford Happiness Questionnaire (1989). Pearson correlation coefficient and T-test were used to analyse data. They found that emotional intelligence, happiness, and mental health are positively related.

A study by Hafen et al. (2011) has explored the relationships among the big five personality traits (agreeableness, neuroticism, openness, conscientiousness, and extraversion), emotional intelligence, and happiness.

The participants were 205 (51 females, 154 males) university students in India. Whether emotional intelligence mediated the relationship between personality traits and feelings of happiness was examined by a series of mediational path analyses. It was found by the analysis that emotional intelligence mediates relationships between several personality factors and happiness in the case of females but not happiness in the case of males for whom it makes an independent contribution to happiness.

CONCLUSION

An exploratory study investigated how people with chronic illness remain happy in spite of the suffering they go through. It was explored as to happiness of these people is shaped by occupational stress and, psychological resources viz; spirituality, emotional intelligence, resilience and different coping styles. 200 middle aged men (aged between 55 to 65 years) participated in the study. All of them were working and married with children. Among the 200 men 100 men were not suffering from any chronic illness and were not under any medication. Among the rest 50 each were suffering from diabetes type (II) and coronary heart disease (CHD) respectively and were all undermedication prescribed by medical practitioners. Hierarchical regression analysis was applied for analysing the data. While emotional intelligence was not found to significantly contribute to happiness of people without any chronic illness the opposite was true for people suffering from chronic illness (diabetes type II or CHD). Coping on the other hand was found to affect happiness in both groups significantly.

The significance of emotional intelligence for the happiness of chronically ill individuals can be explained as follows. Diabetes self-care and the lifelong medical care needed for the disease is burdensome, frustrating, and overwhelming for many patients (Knoll et al., 2006). The ever present threat of complications may disturb social relationships, and adjustment to the disease is accompanied by negative emotions such as anger, isolation, permission, and denial etc. (Cox et al., 1992; Hanson et al., 1995; Goleman, 1995). The literature shows that people with high emotional intelligence can be more successful in managing and, solving emotional problems and, hence manage stress better and lead positive and productive family and social lives (Mathews et al., 2000). It is quite possible that emotional intelligence in diabetic patients help them to cope better with negative emotions raised by the illness and experience more positive affects leading to happiness. Emotional intelligence also promotes better social relationships and helps, in turn to build a better social support network, which gives rise to well-being and happiness. Moreover, the literature also shows that perceived ability to use, manage and express emotions and frequent experience of positive emotions is associated with decreased severity of CHD (Panagiotakos et al., 2002; O'Donnell and Elosua, 2008). This probably explains why emotional intelligence contributes positively to the happiness of CHD patients.

Coping was found to be predicting happiness of diabetic patients significantly. Diabetic patients have to adjust with their disease originated physical problems. Naturally self-care as well as responding to treatments gives rise to prolonged distress. Coping helps them to deal with the problems arising from the illness effectively. So, the illness if coped properly does not create stress. As a result, negative emotions arising because of stress can be avoided to experience more positive affects for a happy life. Because according to a study by Lyubomirsky et al. (2005) positive affect facilitate happiness.

The findings of the present study accept the hypothesis that proper coping and emotional intelligence are indeed very essential for a happy life in the case of chronic illness. The study deals with middle aged men and shows how the negative effects of chronic illness can be overcome. Researches reveal that middle-aged people are vulnerable to chronic illnesses.

At the same time this phase of life is full of responsibilities. Therefore, ways in which effective coping and proper emotional handling can be undertaken should be the concern in midlife. Health promoting lifestyles such as exercise, meditation, and yoga which are considered to give mental strength and emotional balance should be practiced. Emotional intelligence is found to be trainable by some researchers. Therefore, promoting these training facilities can be a positive step towards fighting effects of chronic illness.

Researches in this field are needed to pinpoint the psychological resources whose augmentation can enhance happiness, arguably the ultimate objective of life.

REFERENCES

Albrecht, G.L. and Devlieger, P.J. (1999). The disability paradox: High quality of life against all odds. *Social Science & Medicine*, 48(8): 977–988.

Ara, M.R. (2013). Emotional intelligence as a predictor of happiness among students. *Academia: An International Multidisciplinary Research Journal*, 3(2) (Nov).

Babamiri, M., Vatankhah, M., Karami Rad, B. and Ghasemi, M. (2014). Relationship between Stress Coping Styles, Negative Automatic Thoughts, Life Quality and Happiness in Hospitalized Cardiovascular Patients. *Jentashapir Journal of Health Research*, 5(2):27–35.

Brackett, M.A. and Mayer, J.D. (2003). Convergent, discriminant, and incremental validity of competing measures of emotional intelligence. *Personality and Social Psychology Bulletin*, 29(99):1147–1158.

Chan, Y.K. and. Lee, R.P.L. (2006). Network size, social support, and happiness in later life: a comparative study of Beijing and Hong Kong. *Journal of Happiness Studies*, 7:87–112.

Charmaz, K. (1983). Loss of self: A fundamental form of suffering in the chronically ill. *Sociology of Health & Illness*, 5(2): 168–195.

Clausen, J.A. (1993). *American lives: Looking back at the children of the Great Depression*. New York: The Free Press.

Cox D.J. and Gonder-Frederick L. (1992). Major developments in behavioural diabetes research. *Journal of Consulting and Clinical Psychology*, 60: 628–638.

Csikszentmihalyi, M., Rathunde, K., Whalen, S. and Wong, M. (1993). *Talented teenagers: The roots of success and failure*. London: Cambridge University Press. 22–23.

Diener, E. (2000). Subjective well-being- the science of happiness and a proposal for a national index. *American Psychologist*, 55(1): 34–43.

Duval, M.L. (1984). Psychosocial metaphors of physical distress among MS patients. *Social Science & Medicine*, 19(6): 635–638.

Felton, B.J. and Revenson, T.A. (1984). Coping with chronic illness: A study of illness controllability and the influence of coping strategies on psychological adjusts. *Journal of Counseling and Clinical Psychology*, 52: 343–353.

Franklin, S.S. (2010). *The Psychology of Happiness A Good Human Life*. Cambridge University Press.

Furnham, A. and Petrides, K.V. (2008). Trait emotional intelligence and happiness. *Emotional intelligence: Perspectives on educational and positive psychology*. In J.C. Cassady, & M.A. Eissa (Eds). New York: Peter Lang. 121–129.

Goleman, D. (1995). *Emotional Intelligence*. New York: Bantam.

Gowing, M.K. (2001). Measurement of emotional competence. *The emotionally intelligent workplace*. In C. Cherniss and D. Goleman (Eds.). San Francisco. CA: Jossey-Bass. 83–131.

Hafen, C.A., Singh, K. and Laursen, B. (2011). The happy personality in India: The role of emotional intelligence. *Journal of Happiness Studies. October*. Vol. 12, Issue 5: 807–817.

Hanson, C.L., de Guire, M.J., and Schinkel, A.M. (1995). Empirical validation for a family-centered model of care. *Diabetes Care*, 18:1347–1356.

Hoppe, S. (2013). Chronic illness as a source of happiness paradox or completely normal. *Health, Culture and Society*, 5(1).

Kamen-Siegel, L., Rodin, J., Seligman, M.E.P. and Dwyer, J. (1991). Explanatory style and cell- mediated immunity in elderly men and women. *Health Psychology*, 10(4): 229-235.

Knoll, M.J., Twisk, J.W., Beekman, A.T.F., Heine, R.J. Snoek, F.J. and Pouwer, F. (2006). Depression as a risk factor for the onset of type 2 diabetes mellitus: A meta-analysis. *Diabetologia*, 49(5):837–845.

Koopmans, T.A. and Zitman, G. (2010). Effects of happiness on all-cause mortality during 15 years of follow up: The Arnhem Elderly Study. *Journal of Happiness Studies*, 11(1):113–124.

Koopmanschap, M. (2002). Coping with Type II diabetes: the patient's perspective. *Diabetologia*, 45:S18–S22.

Langenhof, M.R. and Komedur, J. (2018). Why and how the early-life environment affects development of coping behaviours. *Behavioral Ecology and Sociobiology*, 72:34.

Lazarus, R.S. (1974). The psychology of coping: Issues of Research and Assessment *Coping and Adaptation.* In G.V. Coceho, D.A. Humberg and J.E. Adams (eds.). New York: Basic Books.

Lopes, P.N., Salovey, P. and Strauss, R. (2004). Emotional intelligence, personality, and the perceived quality of social relationships. *Personality and Individual Differences*, 35: 641–658.

Lyubomirsky, S., King, L. and Diener, E. (2005). The benefits of frequent positive affect: Does happiness lead to success? *Psychological Bulletin*, 131(6): 803–855.

Marinic, M. and Brkljacic, T. (2008). Love over gold-the correlation of happiness level with some life satisfaction factors between persons with and without physical disability. *Journal of Developmental and Physical Disabilities*, 20(6): 527–540.

Matthews G. and Zeidner M. (2000). *The Handbook of Emotional Intelligence: Theory, Development, Assessment and Application at Home, School and in the Workplace.* Bar-On R, Parker JDA, eds. San Francisco, CA: Jossey-Bass; 459.

Meyers, A.R. (2000). From function to felicitude: Physical disability and the search for happiness in health services research. *American Journal of Mental Retardation*, 105(5): 342–351.

Mowrer, O.H. (1960). *Learning Theory and Behaviour.* New York: Wiley.

Navrady, L.B., Zeng, Y., Clarke, T.K., Adams, M.J., Howard, D.M., Deary, L.J. and McIntosh, A.M. (2018). Genetic and environmental contributions to psychological resilience and coping. *Welcome Open Research*, 3: 12.

Newman, S., Fits Patrick, R., Lamb, R. and Shiplay, M. (1990). Patterns of coping in rheumatoid arthritis. *Psychological and Health*, 4: 187–200.

O'Donnell, C.J. and. Elosua, R. (2008). Cardiovascular risk factors. Insights from Framingham Heart Study. *Revista Española de Cardiología*, 61(3): 299–310.

Pahuja, Y., Khan, S.M. and Pestonjee, D.M. (2016). The effects of occupational stress and emotional intelligence on individual happiness– Causal Analysis. *International Journal of Social Science and Economics Invention*, 2(2): 1–12.

Panagiotakos, D.B., Pitsavos, C., Chrysohoou, C., Stefanadis, C. and Toutouzas, P. (2002). Risk stratification of coronary heart disease in Greece: Final results from the CARDIO2000 Epidemiological Study. *Preventive Medicine*, 35(6): 548–556.

Paranjpe, A.C., and Rao, K.R. (2008). Psychology in the Advita Vedanta. *Handbook of Indian Psychology*. In K.R. Rao, A.C. Paranjpe, and A.K. Dalal (Eds.). New Delhi: Cambridge University Press. 253–285.

Rojas, M. (2005). A conceptual- referent theory of happiness: Heterogenity and its consequences. *Social Indicators Research*, 74(2): 261–294.

Ruiz-Aranda, D., Extremera, N. and Pineda-Galán, C. (2014). Emotional intelligence, life satisfaction and subjective happiness in female student health professionals: The mediating effect of perceived stress. *Journal of Psychiatric and Mental Health Nursing*, 21(2):106–113.

Saha, S., Chakraborty, D. and Chaudhuri, A. (2015). Happiness and Its contributory factors: A study on urban youth population. *Indian Journal of Positive Psychology*, 6(4): 397–400.

Salagame, K.K.K. (2015). Indian perspective and positive psychology. *Positive Psychology Application in Work, Health, and Well-Being*. In Kumar, U., Archana and Parkash, V (Eds). Pearson India Education Services Pvt. Ltd.

Salovey, P. and Mayer, J.D. (1990). Emotional intelligence. *Imagination, Cognition, and Personality*, 9: 185–211.

Sasanpour M., Khodabakhshi M. and Nooryan, K.H. (2012). The relationship between emotional Intelligence, Happiness and Mental Health in Students of Medical Sciences of Isfahan University.

International Journal of Collaborative Research on Internal Medicine & Public Health, 4(9): 1614.

Segerstrom, S.C., Taylor, S.E., Kemeny, M.E. and Fahey, J.L. (1998). Optimism is associated with mood, coping, and immune change in response to stress. *Journal of Personality and Social Psychology,* 74:1646–1655.

Seligman, M.E.P. and Csikszentmihalyi, M. (2000). Positive psychology: An introduction. *American Psychologist*, 55: 5–14.

Singh, J.K. (2015). Progress in positive psychology: Some reflections from India. *Positive psychology Application in work, health, and well-being.* In Kumar.U, Archana and Parkash, V (Eds). Pearson India Education Services Pvt. Ltd.

Snyder, C.R., Lopez, S.J. and Pedrotti, J.T. (2011). *Positive Psychology: The Scientific and Practical Exploration of Human Strength.* Second edition. Sage Publications.

Stewart, D.C. and Sullivan, T.J. (1982). Illness behavior and the sick role in chronic disease: The case of multiple sclerosis. *Social Science & Medicine,* 16(15): 1397–1404.

Taylor, D.W. (2010). *The Burden of Non-Communicable Diseases in India.* The Cameron Institute. Hamilton.

Thorne, S. and Paterson, B. (1998). Shifting images of chronic illness. *Image: The Journal of Nursing Scholarship*, 30(2): 173–178.

Veenhoven, R. (1997). The utility of happiness. *Social Indicators Research,* 20:333–354.

Wethington, E. (2003). Turning points as opportunities for psychological growth. *Flourishing: Positive Psychology and the life well-lived.* In C.L. M. Keys and J. Haidt (Eds.), Washington, D.C.: American Psychological Association.

WHO (2005). *Preventing Chronic Diseases: A Vital Investment: WHO Global Report.* World Health Organization.

In: A Socio-Economic and Demographic ...   ISBN: 978-1-53619-023-6
Editors: A. Rodriguez Andres et al.   © 2021 Nova Science Publishers, Inc.

Chapter 4

COLLEGE MENTAL HEALTH IN INDIA: COPING WITH A POTENTIAL CRISIS

Rajlakshmi Guha[*]
Centre for Educational Technology
Indian Institute of Technology, Kharagpur, India

ABSTRACT

College is a time for exploring new interests and sources of knowledge and experiencing the new found autonomy of adulthood. Yet stress can mark this transition to adulthood with increased expectations from self and others, potential financial worries, uncertainties about the future, and apprehensions about old and new relationships. Often the student's inability to cope with the mentioned stressors impacts academic success and social interactions with potential implications for mental health and overall wellbeing. The consequences vary from anxiety and depression to substance abuse. Reliable data points to an alarming increase in the global incidence of mental health disorders among college students. India, with the largest youth population in the world, is at risk of

---

[*] Corresponding Author's E-mail: rajlakshmiguha@gmail.com.

being hugely affected over the next 20 years unless corrective measures are taken; data provided by college mental health services support such apprehensions. On the basis of secondary and primary data, this paper identifies the triggers for mental health problems among college going youth and suggests ways to check their incidence and prevalence.

Keywords: college students, mental health disorder, well-being

INTRODUCTION

College life is one of the most aspired and cherished moments of youth. College gives the student an opportunity to explore deeper sources of knowledge. In college the student selects his preferred subject of choice and thus can delve deeper into the subject, not restricted by syllabi. The college years are also representative of a new found autonomy that was inaccessible during the school years.

College life is associated with the emergence of several factors that influence an individual's development and personality. The college community is an environment in which the student conducts his daily activities, in the process interacting with peers, seniors and professors intimately and personally (Siggins, 2010). This community plays a very significant role in the crucially important phase of personal development that occurs during the college years.

Mental health problems are very common among college students (Blanco, 2008). Kessler et al. (2007) observed that 75% of individuals who experience a mental disorder during their lifetime are struck by its first onset by 25 years of age. Symptoms of a mental illness may affect a student at any point of his career. Mental illness can be acute or chronic. It is important for institutions to be aware that not all mental health difficulties constitute a 'disability'. To a significant extent, this awareness exists among the administration of educational institutions and their regulators. Thus, mental health problems do not necessarily prevent an individual from carrying out his academic responsibilities. This indicates that there are a large number of students who develop mental health problems and also continue with college education during this age. Thus, the college years represent a crucial period with regard to mental health and health behaviours.

The increase of mental health problems and disorders among college goers and the subsequent absence of a standardized framework for dealing with college mental health in India is an emerging concern. The incorporation of mental health services in the development of an integrated policy for addressing mental health in Indian college settings is of utmost necessity.

This chapter attempts to describe the factors affecting mental health of college goers and provide the reader an idea of the prevalence of mental health disorders in college students. It then elaborates on the specific mental health disorders that are prevalent during these college years and the importance of early identification of mental health disorders in students as well as the development of outreach strategies. Finally, it touches upon the existing policies for college mental health in India and as a use case discusses an existing framework to address mental health needs in a residential college setting in India.

CAUSES OF MENTAL HEALTH DISORDERS DURING COLLEGE LIFE

Individuals at this stage of life are at a transition to adulthood and all the responsibilities that come along with it. This transitional stage inevitably involves specific developmental changes. Many individuals are, as a consequence of these changes, afflicted by psychological disturbances during this phase which cause irreversible damage to their lives. It is thus important to comprehend the risk factors affecting mental health during this period, with an emphasis on improving mental health outcomes for college students.

NEUROBIOLOGICAL DEVELOPMENT DURING COLLEGE YEARS

Morphological evidence along with neurobehavioral and neurochemical research suggests that the brain remains under construction during adolescence (Giedd et al., 1999; Wahlstrom et al., 2010; Kaplan, 2004). Sowell et al. (1999, 2001) suggested a significant reduction of gray matter density from childhood to adolescence and from adolescence to young adulthood. Cognitive, emotional, and social implications are an integral part of maturation and development during young adulthood.

Magnetic resonance imaging (MRI) research reports that the neuro-circuitry remains structurally and functionally vulnerable during this age and myelinogenesis continues during the college years. Due to the marked increases in sex hormones (progesterone, estrogen, and testosterone) during puberty and its interaction with environmental input, various physiological parameters like eating and sleeping habits, and sexual behaviour are influenced. The limbic system also undergoes significant changes during this developmental period which likewise has an impact on decision-making and problem-solving ability, novelty seeking and risk-taking behaviours, impulsivity and self-control, and outward emotional expressions. The prefrontal cortex develops last during brain maturation and the executive functions of the prefrontal cortex remain under developed. This explains why many college students display immature behaviour.

During this post adolescence period, the neuro-circuitry strengthens, and functions like the ability to process complex information, multitasking and problem-solving behaviours improve.

Brain plasticity also provides an opportunity to develop talents and personal interests during this age. However, several factors like trauma or insult, substance abuse, chronic stress, and sedentary lifestyles may have a negative impact on this developmental period of brain maturation (Dahl, 2003; Blakemore, 2012).

STRESS AND COLLEGE LIFE

Indian movies more often than not represent college as a fun-filled place with joy and comforts. Unfortunately, college life also has its stressors for students. College goers experience a large number of stressors including academic issues, financial concerns, and/or social strains (Skowron et al., 2004). Causes of stress during college that have been well documented deal with exams and assignments, the pressure for completion of project deadlines and of competition, peer and parental pressure, and inability to concentrate (Kitzrow, 2009; Sher, 1996; Gallagher, 2000; O'Malley, 1990; Stone, 1990). The stressors may also result from challenges arising from procrastination, problems with interpersonal relationships, or fear of academic failure.

In the Indian scenario, most of the students going to vocational institutes for higher education also carry the burden of a financial loan. Pressure to succeed, acquire a good job at the end of college life and meet societal approval; concerns regarding future uncertainties; along with social and emotional issues related to relationships are often causes of worry and stress. In India, students joining premier institutes for engineering and medical studies have to clear a highly competitive entrance examination that entails grooming and preparation for more than four years. Thus, these students have the additional burden of maintaining their academic excellence demonstrated by their clearing the mentioned entrance exams. More often than not, these students are usually high achievers and have excelled in academics throughout their lives, being high performers in their local schools, village/ city or states. Joining a premier institute puts them amidst other toppers across the country. Thus, many of these past toppers obviously and suddenly find themselves not at the top of the class, a new experience which challenges the positive self-images of 'being toppers' experienced since childhood. Given that this stage of life entails consolidation of personal identity along with academic and sexual identity, such self-doubt and inner conflict often gives way to further stress. Several of my own students have complained of the incongruity and pain resulting from a dual existence – a person who is not a good performer in college who simultaneously, as a result of social pressures, has to live up to the image of the 'high achiever' that others have of him in the home environment. A large number of students studying in premier academic institutes in India often try and avoid home environment to ward-off these stressors.

Underlying risk factors for mental health issues vary from person to person and are not always directly related to their college experiences. Nevertheless, particular aspects of the academic experience and environment may cause excessive stress to some students. Transition phases in life can be challenging and act as stressors - like the onset of a new academic environment at the start of the college years. Most students adapt well to their changing environments and lifestyle.

In India, students travel the length and breadth of the country to study in higher academic institutions of repute. Most of the students report of adjustment issues soon after joining the Institution. India having a large diversity in culture, climate, language and food habits, many students face problems in adjusting to the new environment and coping with the associated academic stressors along (Das and Bhattacharya, 2015).

It is important to note that stress does not necessarily have to have a negative impact but may act as a stimulator that enhances performance. Not all students deal with stress ineffectively. Some students take the stressors as a challenge and increase productivity, aiming for higher goals in life. But a large number of students succumb to the stressors and often manifest psychological symptoms or illnesses during the college years.

PREVALENCE OF MENTAL HEALTH ISSUES AMONG COLLEGES GOERS IN WORLD

In recent years, there has been an increase in reported symptoms of mental illnesses in college student populations. An epidemiological study demonstrated that mental health diagnoses among college students have risen from 22% to 36% between 2000 and 2009 (Brownson, 2010). A survey of directors of college counselling centres in the United States of America reveals that 94% of these directors report an increase in incidence of mental illness among students of their institutions. (Gallagher, 2015). The ACHA-NCHA (American College Health Association, 2019) also reports increasing numbers of serious mental health problems. However, a part of this increase in numbers could be a more permissive environment resulting in a greater proportion of students with mental health problems going in for counselling or seeking other medical help.

The All India Survey for Higher Education (AISHE) (2018-19) states that there are 993 enlisted Universities, 39931 Colleges and 10725 Stand Alone Institutions. The total number of registered students in higher educational institutions is approximately 37.4 million with 19.2 million males and 18.2 million females.

According to a study by the World Health Organization for Care of Mental Health (WHO, 2019), India tops the list of countries in regard to the burden of mental and behavioural disorders. Mental illness is a significant public health challenge in India. Several meta-analytic studies of epidemiological variables measuring the incidence of mental disorders in India, estimate the prevalence at between 5.82% (Reddy and Chandrashekar, 1998) and 7.3% (Ganguli, 2000). The National Mental Health Survey of India conducted in 2014-15 (Gururaj et al., 2018), reported a lifetime prevalence rate of mental disorders of 13.7%,, and indicated that nearly 150 million Indians currently require active intervention. A study reporting counselling services in a residential college in India (Das and Bhattacharya, 2015) stated that roughly 2% of students reported to the Counselling Centre for assistance.

TYPES OF MENTAL DISORDERS PREVALENT AMONG COLLEGE STUDENTS

Mental health difficulties, often preceded by major life events such as a bereavement, financial loss, end of a relationship, or loss of career opportunities, can impact significantly on how students perceive themselves and their lives. Symptoms of mental illness may affect anyone at any time, resulting in physiological and mental conditions that can interfere with the student's college experience and with implications for her academic performance.

As mentioned, the increase in incidence of mental illness over time, as reported by surveys or databases, may not necessarily be a true representation of the increase in prevalence of mental illness in a college setting, but rather a representation of how help seeking behaviour amongst students has changed. In the absence of consistent longitudinal data on disorders across student populations in India, it is difficult to understand the changing trends suggested.

The most prevalent mental disorder amongst the youth are anxiety disorders and approximately 11.9% of students suffer from them during their college years (Blanco, 2008). Social phobia has an early age of onset (between 7– 14 years), while panic disorder, generalized anxiety disorders (GAD), and post-traumatic stress disorder (PTSD) usually have later onsets (Kessler, 2005). PTSD usually peaks between the ages of 16 to 17 years, with approximately 33% of a sample developing the disorder by 14 years of age (Giaconia, 1994). Subramaniam et al. (2012) examined 6,616 respondents and reported that the mean age of onset for obsessive compulsive disorder (OCD) was 19 years and 20 years for GAD.

The feeling of anxiety generally is characterized as diffuse and unpleasant with a sense of apprehension or worry, muscle tension, perspiration, restlessness, headache, and chest and stomach discomfort. In a college setting most of the common problems that students report to a counselling center are features of anxiety (Das and Bhattacharya, 2015). Anxiety can produce memory problems, confusion and cognitive distortions. Anxiety becomes a disorder when the symptoms are severe, pervasive, and persistent, and they interfere with daily functioning. Anxiety disorders can develop very quickly or gradually over long periods of time. Chronic anxiety can sometimes be debilitating and interfere with class attendance, assignment submissions, exam performance, interpersonal relationships, social activities, and other day to day activities in a student's life. Anxiety disorders are not rare and are often comorbid with other disorders. Genetic vulnerability, physiological causes, life events, social contexts, and developmental phases may add to the etiology and expression of pathological anxiety.

Another common mental health problem among college students is depression, with prevalence rates in college students of 7 to 9%. (Gallagher, 2000; Blanco et al., 2008). Depression is estimated to affect 350 million people (Marcus et al., 2012). According to the estimates of the World Health Organization, 322 million people, amounting to 4.4% of the world population, suffer from depression (WHO, 2019). Zisook et al. (2007) found that 50% of all cases of depression had their first onset by young adulthood. In the National Comorbidity Survey Replication study, Kessler et al. (2005) reported that 20% of individuals with depression had their first episode by the age of 25 years. With the ongoing demographic trend, depression will increase to 5.7% of the total burden of the disease and result as the second leading cause of disability adjusted life years (DALYs), second only to ischemic heart disease. By 2030, it is expected to be the largest contributor to the disease burden (Grover et al., 2010; WHO, 2013).

There have been quite a few studies on depression among youth in India but mostly with small samples in diverse populations. There have also been a few studies within the medical community (Taneja et al., 2018; Sarkar et al., 2017; Kumar et al., 2012). In a study of college students, Kumar et al. (2014) found that family history of depression and chronic physical disease are important risk factors of depression in students. They also reported that more than one-third of subjects with depression were dissatisfied with the course of study they were enrolled in and mostly perceived their parents as incompatible with their thought processes.

Bipolar affective disorder (BAD) is another mental illness that has its onset mostly during the college years. In a study by Blanco et al. (2008), approximately 3.2 % of college students were diagnosed with BAD. Literature suggests that at least one-third of adults with BAD have their onset as early as 12 years of age (Perlis et al., 2009).

Completed suicides and attempts are higher in youth with mood disorders as compared to healthy people of the same age group (Brent et al., 1993; Geller et al., 2008). It is important to note that students might pick up vulnerabilities to mental illness before entering college and college life might be the trigger that transforms these vulnerabilities to symptoms.

Suicide is the third leading cause of death among young adults and is a significant problem among college students (CDC, 2013). Every hour one student commits suicide in India, with about 28 such suicides reported every day, according to data compiled by the National Crime Records Bureau (NCRB). The NCRB data reports 10,159 student deaths by suicide in 2018, an increase from 9,905 in 2017, and 9,478 in 2016. A random sample collected over 15 universities across USA (Downs et al, 2012) reported that among 8,487 students, 6.7 % stated that they had suicidal ideation, 1.6 % reported as having a suicide plan, and 0.5 % reported making a suicide attempt in the past year. Most students with suicidal ideations and intent do not seek help and this emerges as a serious concern in regard to college mental health, considering the large number of students lost to suicide (Kisch et al., 2005; Drum et al., 2009). Among the major risk factors for suicide in this age group are fallouts in relationships, family issues, depression (Farabaugh, 2012), hopelessness (Dougherty et al., 2009; Rujescu et al., 2012), and substance use (Cash et al., 2009; Bridge et al., 2006).

The lifetime prevalence of depression, anxiety, and stress among adolescents and young adults globally is estimated as 5% to 70%, with variation by study area and over time. In the Indian context, a study by Sahoo et al. (2010) of young adults in the city of Ranchi, Jharkhand, reported that depressive symptoms were present in 18.5% of the population, anxiety in 24.4%, and stress in 20% of young adults. Clinical depression was present in 12.1% and generalized anxiety disorder in 19.0%. The study showed comorbid symptoms to be high - 87% of those having depression also suffered from anxiety disorder. Detecting depressive symptoms, anxiety features, and other stressors detrimental to mental health are essential as it can help stop many individuals from attempting suicide or ending their life in despair.

Another major concern that acts as a stressor and/or a trigger for mental health issues during college life today is the increase in alcoholism and substance use during the college years. Substance use and abuse have been a rising concern globally and in India. Substance abuse is any maladaptive pattern of substance use leading to clinically significant distress or impairment in occupational and social functioning and in the students' life as well as his academic performance. Students abusing substances generally express the inability to control the use of the substance or abstain from the substance. Many students shift from one substance to the other in an attempt to quit use. Substance use and abuse is often closely associated with the development of serious withdrawal symptoms after cessation of or reduction in use.

Alcohol, tobacco, and cannabis are the commonly used substances by young adults but the use of hard drugs like cocaine and LSD is not unheard of in Indian colleges. Increasing use of substances lead to the possibility of a large repertoire of mental health issues, primarily substance induced mood disorders.

In India, the incidence of alcohol use ranges from 3.8% to 21.0%, with men 9.7 times more likely to regularly use alcohol as compared to women (Goel et al., 2015). About 2.8% of the population (31 million individuals) reports having used a cannabis product within the previous year. Incidence of smoking in youth has been estimated at 19.0% in males and 8.3% in females. A transition from smoking tobacco to cannabis is often observed among college goers. The use of cannabis is of two broad types: the legal form (*bhang*) and other illegal cannabis products (*ganja* and *charas*). Around 0.55% of Indians receive support for opioid use problems (Report of Ministry of Social Justice and Empowerment, GOI, 2019). Recreational drug use has become more popular and may be a representative behaviour of the youth, thus, increasing the need to monitor drug use trends, especially among college going students.

Eating disorders, such as bulimia, anorexia, and binge eating are common in the western culture and often have their onset during adolescence with a rapid increase in risk during early adulthood (Hudson et al., 2007). This disorder was not a very common occurrence in the Indian schools or colleges even a few years ago. With global acculturation and an increasing concern over body image and need for acceptance, eating disorders are becoming a significant concern in the urban colleges of India (Nivedita et al., 2018). Bulk of the burden of the incidence of *Anorexia Nervosa* in the age group of 15–19 years is borne by females, with males accounting for only 20% of the incidence. The prevalence rate has increased from 1990 to 2016 (Mohandoss, 2016).

Attention-deficit/hyperactivity disorder (ADHD) is yet another mental health disorder that is of serious concern during the college years. Academic demands require an individual to focus and persevere for long hours. Inattentiveness often leads to poor academic performance and may in itself become a stressor for the individual. ADHD onsets during childhood and persists into adulthood in approximately 50% of cases and negatively affects many critical areas of the life of young adults. Between 2 and 8 % of college students suffer from ADHD (DuPaul et al., 2009). ADHD is associated with poor academic performance (Biederman et al., 2009), social difficulties, and an increased risk for alcohol and drug use (Green et al., 2012) that further exacerbates academic and social difficulties in college. Though with increasing age the hyperactivity in ADHD patients reduces, impulsivity is a common feature during young adulthood and leads to several novelty seeking behaviour, resulting in in a large number of accidents.

Jaisoorya et al. (2019) studied ADHD retrospectively in 5784 college students in India and found that individuals reporting ADHD symptoms in childhood had a higher probability of alcohol and tobacco use, emotional distress, suicidal thoughts and attempts, and poor academic performance. Jhambh (2014) highlighted that ADHD is prevalent even among the college students studying in the most competitive institutes. Students with ADHD experience poorer self-esteem than others and higher emotional instability. Prompt detection and management of ADHD in college students may help them deal with these problems effectively.

One of the most serious mental disorders affecting the youth is Schizophrenia. The average age of onset for men and women is 18 and 25 years respectively. Patients suffering from schizophrenia need emergent medical attention and thus it is important for academic institutions to comprehend the immenseness of the burden of the disease. A student suffering from schizophrenia may develop delusions of grandiosity or persecution and be mostly considered as 'strange' or 'weird' by fellow peers without being reported unless the condition is truly debilitating. Being closely associated with an institute's counselling centre, I have come across many cases of schizophrenia: examples include several students who had limited their dietary intake to chips and soft drinks, for fear of being poisoned by fictitious enemies lurking behind the walls. A few also reported of being watched night and day through hidden cameras placed within the room confines. Unfortunately, students suffering from Schizophrenia or other psychotic disorders get reported long after the onset of illness. This highlights the importance of the various units of an academic institution working in close alliance for the detection and management of mental health issues among students.

There is a paucity of literature regarding the prevalence of schizophrenia among college students in India; however, it appears that symptoms in the psychotic spectrum are not uncommon among college students. Sham et al. (1994) studied 270 schizophrenic probands and found a rapid increase in the onset of schizophrenia in late teens and early twenties. Similar results were found by Hafner et al. (1993). This implies that young adults in college may experience the prodromal phase or the first onset of a psychotic disorder and with a stress diathesis, the probability of getting affected increases during this age.

Another important concern during the college years is the emergence of behavioural addictions. With the increase of computer and internet use, a large number of students suffer from pathological internet dependence (Goel et al., 2013). An exploratory study undertaken by Nair (2006) reported pathological internet dependency in 36.67 per cent of the students. Unpublished data from the counselling centre at Indian Institute of Technology, Kharagpur indicates that almost 10% of the students requiring counselling services have pathological internet dependency.

Mental health issues during college affect the student's academic performance and also have implications for his future, beyond the college years. Substance abuse and mental illnesses are closely associated with negative outcomes ranging from unemployment, financial problems, and future social relationships (Jennison, 2004; Arria et al., 2013; Hasler et al., 2005). This underlines the importance of prompt and adequate treatment of psychopathology to prevent neurocognitive and functional decline. It is thus essential for college administration to focus on these factors for an integrated well-being program for the institute.

Significance of Early Identification of Mental Health Problems and Outreach Strategies

The burden of mental illness is rising at a catastrophic rate. An identification of causal factors has helped in the design of plans and policies. However, it has been estimated that the resources on college campuses are insufficient for the implementation of these policies. The treatment gap, measured as the proportion of individuals affected by a disorder that remain untreated, is very high (Thirunavukarasu, 2011). It is well established that nearly 66% of individuals with a diagnosed mental disorder never seek help from health professionals (Luthra, 2017). Within the student population, where mental illness is associated with a significant stigma and considered by many as a sign of weakness, the eagerness to seek clinical help is lower.

Mental health problems not being identified, often resulting from students and their families living in denial of symptoms characterizing mental illness and not seeking help, contribute significantly to the magnitude of mental health problems in India. One of the major issues that affects diagnosis and treatment of a mental illness is the lack of awareness amongst the population that it is treatable just like physical illnesses. The stigma attached to mental health is also an important concern, especially amongst students.

This burden is enhanced by the lack of facilities available within close reach. This issue has been addressed with the initiative of the Ministry of Human Resource Development (MHRD), Government of India by setting up College mental health units as an essential service in all Centrally Funded Technological Institutes in India. This included some of the premier institutions of India, namely the Indian Institutes of Technology (IITs), Indian Institutes of Management (IIMs), and National Institutes of Technology (NITs).

This response by MHRD has helped to reach out to a large number of residential college students across the country. Some of the IITs have regular counselling centres with clinical staff employed while some of the institutions have outsourced the services to agencies that assist them in addressing students' mental health needs. Despite the availability of a counselling centre within college campus and stigma gradually giving way to acceptance, a large number of students still hesitate to avail services due to the taboo attached to mental health. This is corroborated by Zivin et al. (2009) in their study, through which they found that more than 50% of students with mental health issues persisting over a period of 2 years did not receive treatment as they did not seek help. Most of the barriers to help-seeking in student population include privacy concerns, lack of emotional openness, lack of time, and a belief that one can deal with a mental health problem without clinical assistance. This belief more often than not is also shared by the larger environment including parents and society who feel that engaging in a disciplined lifestyle shall help deal with the disorder better than clinical adherence.

The problem of low treatment seeking in college students may be addressed by the use of technology. Several Indian institutes have introduced the online mode of counselling, which preserves anonymity, for students. Most of these resources are outsourced by the institutions and supplement the provision of physical and mental health service within campus. Escoffery et al. (2005) in their study found that 74 % of the students received health information online, and more than 40 % reported that they sought health information from the internet.

EXISTING POLICIES FOR COLLEGE MENTAL HEALTH IN INDIA

The Mental Health Care Act 2017 (Government of India, 2017) offers comprehensive mandates and guidelines for mental health services in India and explicitly mentions the rights of adults and minors seeking mental healthcare in the country.

The National Youth Policy 2014, Ministry of Youth Affairs and Sports, Govt. of India, identifies

1. psychological and emotional disorders as a youth-specific issue requiring a focused approach
2. the impact of substance use and the risk of depression and suicides amongst the youth and highlights the importance of addressing these issues
3. the short-term and long-term indicators of the impact of psychological and emotional disorders

This policy has made relevant contributions to emphasize the importance of catering to the mental health of the country's youth.

The United Nations 2030 Agenda for Sustainable Development (Goal 3), points out the significance of mental health and wellbeing, and aims to ensure health and wellbeing for all individuals across all age groups including adolescents and youth. It identifies the prevalence of mental disorders, with emphasis on depression and anxiety-related disorders, as a cause of suicide. It also identifies substance use and substance use disorders as a major health concern. India along with several other countries signed the agreement and plans a way forward for the attainment of these goals. However, the national review report on the implementation of the SDGs in India does not mention guidelines for addressing mental health issues.

While all these policies identify the significance of adolescent and youth mental health in some way, India still lacks a comprehensive document focusing on adolescent and youth mental health, and implementation plans for the same.

The establishment of mental healthcare units is a necessity more than a luxury in the current crises in regard to the mental health of Indian youth. Substance use prevention programmes are needed to protect the youth. These should extend beyond the awareness programmes in regard to the dangers of using drugs.

The Ministry of Social Justice and Empowerment, GOI, 2019 has highlighted the importance of prevention programmes for addressing risks associated with substance use and ensuring the safe transience to adulthood, thereby enabling the youth to realize their potential and become productive members of their community and society (Report of The Ministry of Social Justice and Empowerment, GOI, 2019).

The surge in student depression and suicide as well as substance abuse on Indian college campuses has triggered off a significant increase in the availability of college mental health services, which however are still inadequate, given the size of India's youth population. Urgent and impactful interventions are still required.

In addition to identification and treatment of mental health disorders, the college mental health units also need to focus on promoting positive mental health amongst students. Many institutions in India and the global scenario are reviewing their current offering for students to ensure it is promoting self-agency, resilience and independence in the academic community, and is not based on a 'deficit' model where only students who reach the crisis point are offered support.

This shall also serve the purpose of eroding the stigma attached to mental health support as only limited to identification and treatment of psychological vulnerabilities. Providing support to the youth to fulfil their potential is not only in the interest of the institution, but also in the interest of society as a whole.

Addressing Mental Health in a Residential Campus: An Example from a College Setting in India

The success of the university's educational mission depends on the health and well-being of students so that emotional baggage distracting their attention is minimized. The mission of the college mental health service, in working with students on this developmental task, is to help the students fulfil the demands of academic and social life and make the best use of their potential. This involves many people working together to help a student in need. Confidentiality and non-disclosure of information about the mental health of students seeking help in regard to mental illnesses is important.

These centres should also supplement diagnosis and management of mental disorders with promotion of positive mental health and well-being. A collaborative relationship between college mental health centres, and physical health services may lead to an increase in identification and referrals for treatment of students with mental health problems.

Mental health issues affect academic performance and social interactions. Thus, it is imperative to foster collaboration between the faculty and students' groups on the one hand and behavioural health services on the other in helping students in distress. This system has been introduced in India with IIT Kharagpur pioneering the clinical model in 2009. The Counselling Centre of this IIT has clinical psychologists, counsellors and a psychiatrist as its regular staff and works closely with the academic unit, social and cultural unit, the career development centre and the institute health centre for the management and rehabilitation of students with mental health issues. There is also a dedicated body of student volunteers or the 'Students Welfare Group' who work with the academic and campus community for sensitizing students in regard to mental health needs. Active sensitization programmes for de-stigmatizing mental health across all quarters have helped increase help seeking behaviour and the number of footfalls in college mental health centres (Das and Bhattacharya, 2015).

In terms of campus interventions, many campuses have adopted screening programmes and stigma-reduction campaigns, but there are limited published reports demonstrating the effectiveness of these programs, and it is often difficult to generalize results across campuses with differing populations and resources. For suicide prevention, the institute staff, students and security along with all other stake holders are trained to act as effective agents. This model has been adopted by many CFTIs across the country. Many of these institutions have also started using Electronic Medical Records (EMRs) for data keeping and management. Adoption of the use of EMRs has been associated with better planning, coordination, support and care of college students. Unfortunately, a large number of colleges and universities across the country are yet to take an initiative regarding mental health.

CONCLUSION

College mental health is an emerging area of concern in India. The rise in mental health problems among college students in India and the subsequent absence of a standardised framework for dealing with it needs to be addressed urgently. The framework should support new policies for implementing sensitization and awareness programmes for mental health in every college setting in the country. In addition, it should involve the setting up of urgently required Counselling Centres and mental health units that work in liaison with academic units within institutions. It is also important to develop a consortium for college mental health within the country for understanding the dynamic issues that give rise to mental health disorders and comprehending the best possible *Standard Operating Procedures* within the cultural frameworks and academic contexts. This may in future be incorporated in the National Mental Health Act. The academic institution should also supplement diagnosis and management of mental disorders with promotion of positive mental health and well-being.

The success of an academic institute's educational mission depends on the health and well-being of students that drive them to achieve their full potential. It is thus imperative for college administration and relevant policy makers in India to attach seriousness to the promotion of mental health among college students.

REFERENCES

AISHE 2018 -19. *All India Survey on Higher Education, 2018-19.* Government of India, Ministry of Human Resource Development, Department of Higher Education, 2019, New Delhi.

American College Health Association. *American College Health Association-National College Health Assessment II: Undergraduate Student Executive Summary Spring 2019.* Silver Spring, MD: American College Health Association; 2019.

Arria, A.M., Caldeira, K.M., Bugbee, B.A., Vincent, K.B. and O'Grady, K.E. (2013). The academic opportunity costs of substance use during college.

Blakemore, S.J. and Robbins, T.W. (2012). Decision-making in the adolescent brain. *Nature Neuroscience*, 15(9): 1184-1191.

Blanco C, Okuda M, Wright C, Hasin DS, Grant BF, Liu SM, Olfson M. (2008). Mental health of college students and their non-college-attending peers: Results from the National Epidemiologic Study on Alcohol and Related Conditions. *Archives of General Psychiatry*, 65(12):1429–37.

Brent D.A., Perper J.A., Moritz G., Baugher M., Roth C., Balach L. and Schweers J. (1994). Stressful life events, psychopathology, and adolescent suicide: a case control study. *Suicide and Life-Threatening Behavior*, 23(3): 179–187.

Bridge, J.A., Goldstein, T.R. and Brent, D.A. (2006). Adolescent suicide and suicidal behavior. *The Journal of Child Psychology and Psychiatry*, 47(3–4):372–394.

Brownson, C. (2010). Conducting research in college and university counselling centers' in Kay, J. and Schwartz, V. (Ed) Mental Health Care in the College Community. John Wiley & Sons Ltd. ISBN: 978-0-470-74618.

Cash S.J. and Bridge, J.A. (2009). Epidemiology of youth suicide and suicidal behaviour. *Current Opinion in Pediatrics*, 21(5):613–619.

CDC. Centre for Disease Control. Violence Prevention. (2013). Available from: http:// www.cdc.gov/violenceprevention/pub/youth_suicide.html

Dahl, R.E. (2003). Beyond raging hormones: the tinderbox in the teenage brain. *Cerebrum*, 5(3):7–22.

Dougherty, D.M., Mathias, C.W., Marsh-Richard, D.M., Prevette, K.N., Dawes, M.A., Hatzis, E.S., Palmes, G., Nouvion S.O. (2009). Impulsivity and clinical symptoms among adolescents with non-suicidal self-injury with or without attempted suicide. *Psychiatry Research*, 169(1):22–27.

Downs, M.F. and Eisenberg, D. (2012). Help seeking and treatment use among suicidal college students. *Journal of American College Health*, 60(2):104–114.

Drum, D.J., Brownson, C., Burton Denmark, A. and Smith, S.E. (2009). New data on the nature of suicidal crises in college students: Shifting the paradigm. *Professional Psychology: Research and Practice*, 40(3): 213–222.

DuPaul, G.J., Weyandt. L.L., O'Dell, S.M. and Varejao, M. (2009). College students with ADHD: Current status and future directions. *Journal of Attention Disorders*, 13(3):234–250.

Escoffery, C., Miner, K.R., Adame, D.D., Butler, S., McCormick, L. and Mendell, E. (2005). Internet use for health information among college students. *Journal of American College Health*, 53(4): 183–188.

Farabaugh, A., Bitran, S., Nyer, M., Holt, D.J., Pedrelli, P., Shyu, I., Hollon, S.D., Zisook, S., Baer, L., Busse, W., Petersen, T.J., Pender, M., Tucker, D.D., Fava, M. (2012). Depression and suicidal ideation in college students. *Psychopathology,* 45(4):228–234.

Gallagher, S. (2000). Philosophical conceptions of the self: implications for cognitive science. *Trends in Cognitive Sciences,* 4(1):14–21.

Gallagher, R.P. (2015) National Survey of College Counseling Centers 2014. Project Report. The International Association of Counseling Services (IACS). Retrieved from: http://dscholarship.pitt.edu/28178/1/survey_2014.

Ganguli, H.C. (2000). Epidemiological findings on prevalence of mental disorders in India. *Indian Journal of Psychiatry*, 42(1):14–20.

Geller, B., Tillman, R., Bolhofner, K. and Zimerman, B. (2008). Child bipolar I disorder: prospective continuity with adult bipolar I disorder; characteristics of second and third episodes; predictors of 8-year outcome. *Archives of General Psychiatry*, 65(10): 1125–1133.

Giaconia, R.M., Reinherz, H.Z., Silverman, A.B., Pakiz, B., Frost, A.K. and Cohen E. (1994). Ages of onset of psychiatric disorders in a community population of older adolescents. *Journal of the American Academy of Child & Adolescent Psychiatry*, 33(5):706–717.

Giedd, J.N., Blumenthal, J., Jeffries, N.O., et al. (1999) Brain development during childhood and adolescence: A longitudinal MRI study. *Nature Neuroscience*, 2(10):861–863.

Goel, D., Subramanyam, A., Kamath, R. (2013). A study on the prevalence of internet addiction and its association with psychopathology in India adolescents. *India Journal of Psychiatry*, 55:140–143.

Goel, D.S. (2011). Why mental health services in low- and middle-income countries are under-resourced, underperforming: An Indian perspective. *National Medical Journal of India*, 24: 94–97.

Grover, S., Dutt, A. and Avasthi, A. (2010). An overview of Indian research in depression. *Indian Journal of Psychiatry*, 52 (1): 178–188.

Häfner, H, Maurer, K., Löffler, W and Riecher-Rössler, A. (1993). The influence of age and sex on the onset and early course of schizophrenia. *The British Journal of Psychiatry*, 162:80–86.

Hasler, G., Pine, D.S., Kleinbaum, D.G., Gamma, A., Luckenbaugh, D., Ajdacic, V., Eich, D., Rössler, W. and Angst, J. (2005). Depressive symptoms during childhood and adult obesity: the Zurich Cohort Study. *Molecular Psychiatry*, 10(9):842–850.

Hudson, J.I., Hiripi, E., Pope, H.G., Jr and Kessler, R.C. (2007). The prevalence and correlates of eating disorders in the National Comorbidity Survey Replication. *Biological psychiatry*, *61*(3), 348–358.

Jaisoorya, T.S., Gowda, G.S., Nair, B.S., Menon, P.G., Rani, A., Radhakrishnan, K.S., Revamma, M., Jeevan, C.R., Kishore, A., Thennarasu, K. and Benegal, V. (2017). Correlates of high-risk and low-risk alcohol use among college students in Kerala, India. *Journal of Psychoactive Drugs*, 50:54–61.

Jennison, K.M. (2004). The short-term effects and unintended long-term consequences of binge drinking in college: a 10-year follow-up study. *American Journal Drug Alcohol Abuse*, 30(3):659–684.

Jhambh, I., Arun, P. and Garg, J. (2014). Cross-sectional study of self-reported ADHD symptoms and psychological comorbidity among college students in Chandigarh, India. *Industrial psychiatry Journal*, 23(2): 111–116.

Kaplan, P.S. (2004). *Adolescence*. Boston, MA: Houghton Mifflin Company.

Kessler, R.C., Berglund, P., Demler, O., Jin, R., Merikangas, K.R. and Walters, E.E. (2005). Lifetime prevalence and age-of-onset distributions of DSM-IV disorders in the National Comorbidity Survey replication. *Archives of General Psychiatry*, 62(7):768.

Kessler, R.C., Amminger, G.P., Aguilar-Gaxiola, S., Alonso, J., Lee, S. and Ustün, T.B. (2007). Age of onset of mental disorders: a review of recent literature. *Current Opinion Psychiatry*, 20(4):359–364.

Kisch, J., Leino, E.V. and Silverman, M.M. (2005). Aspects of suicidal behavior, depression, and treatment in college students: Results from the spring 2000 national college health assessment survey. *Suicide and Life-Threatening Behavior*, 35(1):3–13.

Kitzrow, M.A. (2009). The mental health needs of today's college students: Challenges and recommendations. *NASPA Journal*, 46(4): 646–660.

Sher, K.J., Wood, M.D., Wood, P.K. and Raskin, G. (1996). Alcohol outcome expectancies and alcohol use: A latent variable cross-lagged panel study. *Journal of Abnormal Psychology*, 105(4), 561–574.

Kumar, H., Kaur, N. and Palaha, R. (2014). Prevalence of multiple antibiotic resistant Escherichia coli serotypes in raw sewage of North-Western Punjab, India. *Indian Journal of Medical Microbiology*, 32:468–470.

Kumar, G.S., Jain, A. and Hegde, S. (2012). Prevalence of depression and its associated factors using Beck depression inventory among students of a medical college in Karnataka. *Indian Journal of Psychiatry*, 54(3): 223–226.

Luthra, M. (2017). Depression: Current scenario with reference to India. *Indian Journal of Community Health,* 29(1): 1–4.

Marcus, M.A., Westra, H.A., Eastwood, J.D. and Barnes, K.L. (2019). *Mobilizing Minds Research Group Ministry of Social Justice. Magnitude of substance use in India.* 2019. National Drug Dependence Treatment Centre (NDDTC), All India Institute of Medical Sciences (AIIMS), New Delhi under Ministry of Social Justice, Government of India. 2019.

Mohandoss, A.A. (2018). A study of burden of anorexia nervosa in India-2016. *Journal of Mental Health Human Behavior*, 23:25–32.

National Crime Records Bureau. *Accidental deaths and suicides in India:* (2018). Ministry of Home Affairs, Government of India, New Delhi, India.

Nivedita, N.G., Sreenivasa, T.G.M., Sathyanarayana, R. and Malini, S.S. (2018). Eating disorder: Prevalence in the student population of Mysore, South India. *India Journal Psychiatry*, 60:433–437.

O'Malley, J.M. and Chamot, A.U. (1990). Learning Strategies in Second Language Acquisition. Cambridge, UK: Cambridge University Press.

Perlis, R.H., Smoller, J.W., Ferreira, M.A., McQuillin, A., Bass, N., Lawrence, J., Sachs, G.S., Nimgaonkar, V., Scolnick, E.M., Gurling, H., Sklar, P. and Purcell, S. (2009). A genomewide association study of response to lithium for prevention of recurrence in bipolar disorder. *American Journal of Psychiatry*, 166(6):718–725.

Pradeep, B.S., Gururaj, G., Varghese, M., Benegal, V., Rao, G.N., Sukumar, G.M., et al. (2018) National Mental Health Survey of India, 2016 - Rationale, design and methods. *PLoS ONE* 13(10): e0205096. https://doi.org/10.1371/journal.pone.0205096

Das, R. and Bhattacharya, S.D. (2015). College psychotherapy at an Indian technical education university's student counselling center. *Journal of College Student Psychotherapy*, 29(2): 90–93.

Reddy, V.M. and Chandrashekar, C.R. (1998). Prevalence of mental and behavioural disorders in India: A meta-Analysis. *Indian Journal of Psychiatry*, 40: 149–157.

Rujescu, D. and Giegling, I. (2012). Intermediate Phenotypes in Suicidal Behavior Focus on Personality. In: Dwivedi, Y., editor. *The Neurobiological Basis of Suicide.* Boca Raton (FL).

Sahoo, S. and Khess, C.R.J. (2010). Prevalence of depression, anxiety, and stress among young male adults in India: A dimensional and categorical diagnoses-based study. *The Journal of Nervous and Mental Disease*, 198(12): 901–904.

Sarkar, S., Gupta, R. and Menon, V. (2017). A systematic review of depression, anxiety, and stress among medical students in India. *Journal of Mental Health and Human Behaviour*, 22(2):88–96.

Sham, P.C., MacLean, C.J. and Kendler, K.S. (1994). A typological model of schizophrenia based on age at onset, sex and familial morbidity. *Acta Psychiatrica Scandinavica*, 89(2):135–141.

Siggins, L.D. (2010). Working with the campus community' in Kay, J. and Schwartz, V. (Ed) *Mental Health Care in the College Community.* John Wiley & Sons Ltd. ISBN: 978-0-470-74618-9.

Skowron, E.A., Wester, S.R. and Azen, R. (2004). Differentiation of self-mediates college stress and adjustment. *Journal of Counselling & Development, 82 (1):* 69–78.

Sowell, E.R., Thompson, P.M., Holmes, C.H.J., Jernigan, T.L. and Toga, A.W. (1999). In vivo evidence for post-adolescence from post-adolescent brain maturation in frontal and striatal regions. *Nature Neuroscience*, 2: 859–861.

Sowell, E.R., Thompson, P.M., Tessner, K.D. and Toga, A.W. (2001). Mapping continued brain growth and gray matter development in dorsal frontal cortex: Inverse relationship during post adolescence brain maturation. *The Journal of Neuroscience*, 21: 8819–8829.

Stone, E.F. and Stone, D.L. (1990). Privacy in organizations: Theoretical issues, research findings, and protection strategies. In G. Ferris & K. Rowland (Eds.), *Research in personnel and human resources management,* Vol. 8, (pp. 549-411). Greenwich, CT: JAI Press.

Subramaniam, M., Abdin, E., Vaingankar, J.A. and Chong, S.A. (2012). Obsessive – compulsive disorder: Prevalence, correlates, help-seeking, and quality of life in a multiracial Asian population. *Social Psychiatry and Psychiatric Epidemiology*, 47(12): 2035–2043.

Taneja, N., Sachdeva, S., Dwivedi, N. (2018). Assessment of depression, anxiety, and stress among medical students enrolled in a medical college of New Delhi, India. *Indian Journal of Social Psychiatry*, 34: 157–162.

The Mental HealthCare Act (2017). Available at https://www.indiacode.nic.in/bitstream/123456789/2249/1/A2017-10.pdf.

Thirunavukarau, M. (2011). Closing the treatment gap. *Indian Journal of Psychiatry*, 53:199–201.

Wahlstrom, D., Collins, P., White, T. and Luciana, M. (2010). Developmental changes in dopamine neurotransmission in adolescence: Behavioral implications and issues in assessment. *Brain and Cognition*, 72(1):146–159.

Marcus, M.A., Westra, H.A., Eastwood, J.D., Barnes, K.L. and Mobilizing Minds Research Group. (2012). What Are Young Adults Saying About Mental Health? An Analysis of Internet Blogs. *Journal of Medical Internet Research*, 14(1).

World Health Organization, Global Burden of Disease 2008: 2004 update. *Geneva: World Health Organization.* [Internet]. [cited 2013Nov5]; Available from: http://www.who.int/healthinfo/global_burden_disease/GBD_report_2004 update_full.pdf, (2013).

World Health Organization. Mental Health Atlas 2017. *World Health Organization;* 2019. p. 68. Available from: https://www.who.int/mental_health/evidence/atlas/mental_health_atlas_2017/en/.

Zisook, S., Lesser, I., Stewart, J.W., Wisniewski, S.R., Balasubramani, G.K., Fava, M., Gilmer, W.S., Dresselhaus, T.R., Thase, M.E., Nierenberg, A.A., Trivedi, M.H. and Rush, A.J. (2007). Effect of age at onset on the course of major depressive disorder. *The American Journal of Psychiatry*, 164(10):1539–46.

Zivin, K., Eisenberg, D., Gollust, S.E. and Golberstein, E. (2009). Persistence of mental health problems and needs in a college student population. *Journal of Affective Disorders*, 17(3):180–185.

In: A Socio-Economic and Demographic … ISBN: 978-1-53619-023-6
Editors: A. Rodriguez Andres et al. © 2021 Nova Science Publishers, Inc.

Chapter 5

EXAMINING THE HAPPINESS STIMULATING IMPACTS OF CLOSE RELATIONSHIPS

*Samadrita Saha[1] and Anindita Chaudhuri[2],**
[1]The Neotia University, Sarisha, India
[2]Department of Psychology, University of Calcutta, Kolkata, India

ABSTRACT

Happiness can be explained by a variety of factors: life satisfaction, appreciation of life, moments of pleasure etc. But at a tautological level happiness results from the experiencing of positive emotions. Through an extensive literature review and a primary survey this paper establishes that such positive emotional experiences and therefore happiness can result from close relationships among humans. That is other things remaining the same, those involved in close relationships, based on mutual disclosure and emotional bonding, are happier than others.

---

* Corresponding Author's E-mail: anicaluniv@gmail.com.

Keywords: happiness, emotions, behavior

INTRODUCTION

From Ancient Greeks and Buddhists to modern philosophers and politicians, thinkers have queried the meaning of happiness (McMahon, 2006). There are as many definitions of happiness as the number of people studying happiness. Websters (1994) simply defines it as a) state of well-being characterized by emotions ranging from contentment to intense joy or b) a pleasurable or satisfying experience. Research studies show that our enduring level of happiness (H) is determined by our happiness set point (S), life circumstances (C) (influenced by aspects of temperament and character such as depression and sleep quality) and intentional or voluntary activities (V). Martin Seligman proposed an equation for happiness: $H = S + C + V$ (Seligman, 2002). Further, Lyubomirsky (2008), a prominent researcher in the field of happiness and author of "The How of Happiness", attached percentages to these components. She suggested that our set point, or happiness level determined by birth or genetics, accounts for 50 percent of happiness; circumstances such as marital status, earnings, and looks determine 10 percent; and the remainder of our happiness comes from intentional activities or things we can do to change our happiness level.

The 7th World Happiness Report; was first released in April 2012 in support of a UN High level meeting on "Wellbeing and Happiness: Defining a New Economic Paradigm". That report presented the available global data on national happiness and reviewed related evidence from the emerging science of happiness, showing that the quality of people's lives can be coherently, reliably, and validly assessed by a variety of subjective well-being measures, collectively referred to then and in subsequent reports as "happiness". Each report includes updated evaluations and a range of commissioned chapters on special topics digging deeper into the science of well-being, and on happiness in specific countries and regions. Often there is a central theme. Last year (2019) it focused on happiness and community: how the concept of happiness has been changing over the past dozen years, and how information technology, governance, and social norms influence communities.

A 2018 report concluded that international ranking of migrant happiness was almost identical to that of the native born. This evidence made a powerful case that the large international differences in life evaluations are driven by the differences in how people connect with each other and with their shared institutions and social norms (World Happiness Report, 2019).

Many people believe that we need free choice in order to be happy. However, research on choice has actually turned up some interesting and contradictory data. Some studies have shown that economic development, democratization, and rising social tolerance have increased the extent to which people perceive that they have free choice. This, in turn, has led to higher levels of happiness around the world (Inglehart, 2008).

People who believe that personal choices, rather than fate, control their future, often have a greater appreciation of freedom of choice than those who credit destiny as determining outcomes. The people who don't depend on fate are thought of as having an internal locus of control, while those favoring luck and fate are said to have an external locus of control. For example, if we think of a novelist selling her first book, she could either send the manuscript off and hope for the best or enlist every useful contact and friend of a friend in making sure the manuscript is given a fair read. In the following sections of this present chapter a trial is taken to ascertain the determining factors of "happiness" in context of relationships and its various aspects.

'Persona'- The Mask We Wear Says a Lot on How We Feel: Happiness and Behavior

Lyubomirsky et al. (2006) found that an individual's intentional behavioral strategies can account for as much as 40% of the variance in happiness.

This is important to note, especially for those individuals who might not have the personality variables that predispose them toward happiness, such as high extraversion (Extraversion is a broad personality trait and extroverts are relatively outgoing, gregarious, sociable, and openly expressive) or low neuroticism (individuals who score high on neuroticism are more likely than average to be moody and to experience such feelings as anxiety, worry, fear, anger, frustration, envy, jealousy, guilt, depressed mood and loneliness). People who are neurotic respond worse to stress and are more likely to interpret ordinary situations as threatening. Specifically, in lieu of positive personality traits, engagement in happiness enhancing strategies or happiness inducing behaviors (HIB) has been empirically validated as a means to increase happiness (Lyubomirsky et al., 2006). Importantly, Tkach and Lyubomirsky (2006) strongly believe genetics do not predetermine happiness and that participating in HIB can increase happiness. Thus, any individual can increase happiness by participating in these activities.

Tkach and Lyubomirsky (2006) have identified eight happiness-enhancing strategies in their research: social affiliation, partying and clubbing, mental control, instrumental goal pursuit, passive leisure, active leisure, religion, and direct attempts. While there are many strategies available, they are not all relied on to the same extent. Researchers exploring engagement in such HIB found that the most frequently used behaviors were maintaining friendships, being optimistic, doing random acts of kindness, and exercising (Warner and Vroman, 2011). The same research also found that the least used HIB were forgiving, avoiding worry, practicing spirituality, and meditation. Others have demonstrated that expressing gratitude is also an effective strategy to increase happiness (Senf and Liau, 2013). At the same time, Warner and Vroman (2011) found, that while there were positive associations between HIB and happiness, the connection was only marginally significant. More research, particularly experimental in design, needs to be done in order to determine the relationship between behaviors that are expected to increase happiness and self- reported happiness.

Personality and Happiness Inducing Behaviour (HIB)

Research has also found that personality traits predict not only happiness, but also the use of HIB. For example, Tkach and Lyubomirsky (2006) found that personality traits were related to engagement in their eight strategies to enhance happiness. Specifically, individuals who are high in extraversion were more involved in happiness inducing behaviors compared to those low on this variable. In another study, extraversion and agreeableness were positively correlated with HIB, whereas, neuroticism was negatively correlated with such strategies (Warner and Vroman, 2011). In particular, these researchers found a strong negative correlation between neuroticism and the avoidance of worry. Extraversion and agreeableness were positively correlated with cultivating relationships, expressing gratitude, doing random acts of kindness, being optimistic, and maintaining good physical health. This suggests that the connection between personality factors such as increased extraversion or neuroticism and happiness may be partly mediated by one's participation in happiness inducing behaviors.

GENDER, PERSONALITY, HAPPINESS AND HIB

Researchers have shown that there is a gender difference in personality, in regard to neuroticism. For instance, Albuquerque et al. (2013) discovered that females were significantly more neurotic than males. However, there was no gender difference in regard to extraversion. Their research also extended to gender differences in both positive and negative affect ('affect' here means feelings or mood). Albuquerque et al. (2013) found that although there were no gender differences in positive affect, there were marginally significant findings for negative affect where females score higher than males. Researchers have also demonstrated gender differences in the use and choice of happiness inducing behaviors. For example, Warner and Vroman (2011) found that men and women tended to rely on different HIBs. Specifically, they found that women reported more engagement in nurturing relationships compared to men and that men reported more experiences of flow compared to women. More research must be conducted on gender differences in happiness and not simply on engagement in particular happiness inducing behaviors.

PERSONALITY AND HAPPINESS

Personality traits have frequently been observed to be associated with happiness. It has been suggested that personality traits may lead individuals to experience life in certain ways which, in turn, influences their happiness. However, the exact mechanisms underlying this relationship remain unknown. A very recent study that hypothesized ways in which individuals endorse strategies for achieving happiness (i.e., orientations to happiness: through a life of pleasure, through a life of engagement, or through a life of meaning) mediates the associations that personality traits have with subjective well-being (i.e., satisfaction with life, positive affect, and negative affect). Results indicated that an orientation to meaning in life partially mediated the relationship between extraversion and life satisfaction. In addition, all three orientations to happiness (i.e., pleasure, engagement, and meaning) partially mediated the relationship between extraversion and positive affect (Pollock et al., 2016).

Personality has been found to be more strongly associated with subjective interpretation of happiness in many instances than life circumstances. In part, this might be due to the fact that temperament and other individual differences can influence people's feelings and evaluations of their lives, but also because people's emotions are an inherent part of personality. A study discussed the heritability of "happiness," or that portion of subjective well-being that is due to genetic differences between individuals. The stability of subjective well-being over time is substantial, and this is likely due in part to the stability of personality. Specific personality traits are related to various types of well-being. For example, extroversion appears to be more strongly related to positive emotions, while neuroticism is more related to negative feelings. Although personality is an important correlate of subjective happiness, situations and life circumstances can in some cases have a considerable influence as well. Furthermore, personality can to some degree change over time, and with it, levels of subjective well-being can change (Diener, 2009). Tkach and Lyubomirsky (2006) stated that many associations between individuals' personality and happiness levels are to some extent mediated by the strategies people use to increase their happiness – in particular affiliation, mental control, and direct attempts.

A study explored the relationships among personality, leisure involvement, leisure satisfaction and happiness in a representative sample of Chinese university students (Lu and Hu, 2005). Extraversion and neuroticism were significant predictors of happiness; leisure satisfaction generated incremental effects which were significant but of a lower magnitude than those generated by personality traits.

Recent studies suggested an important role of neuroticism and extraversion as incremental predictors of subjective well-being outcomes. Research has shown that positive cognitions mediated the relation between personality traits and well-being. A study examined the relationship between neuroticism and extraversion, measured as general and group factors, and subjective happiness through a general positivity factor (social relationships, temperament/adaptation, money, society and culture, and *positive* thinking styles) (Lauriola and Iani, 2017). The general positivity factor completely mediated neuroticism-subjective happiness relationships and overlapped with general neuroticism, whilst it partially mediated extraversion-subjective happiness ones. Other paths to happiness involved cheerfulness and enthusiasm. Assertiveness, motor activity level and seeking excitement had a weak relationship with subjective happiness. Gregariousness and friendliness had neither direct nor indirect effects on subjective happiness. Life satisfaction had a twofold role as a component of positivity as well as providing an independent contribution to variance in subjective happiness. Cheerfulness and extraversion made an incremental contribution to variance in subjective happiness.

A paper which contains two studies set out to examine to what extent attributional style, that is about how one explains the causes of events -

internal, stable or global; and personality traits predicted happiness and psychiatric symptoms in a normal, non-clinical, population of young people in their early twenties (Cheng and Furnham, 2001). Attributional style was a significant predictor of happiness and mental health. It was significantly associated with extraversion and neuroticism. The results indicated that optimistic attributional style was a stronger predictor of self-reported happiness than pessimistic attributional style. Extraverts tended to have optimistic explanatory style for positive outcomes whereas neurotics tended to have pessimistic explanatory style for negative outcomes.

Two studies investigated the predictive ability of romantic relationship quality in regard to happiness above and beyond the influence of personality (Demir, 2008). Study 1 (n = 221) showed that romantic relationship quality accounted for 3% of the variance in happiness while controlling for personality. Study 2 showed that emotional security and companionship emerged as the strongest features of romantic relationship quality that predicted happiness. Besides, identity formation also moderated the relationship between relationship quality and happiness such that individuals were happier when they experienced high quality relationships at high levels of identity formation.

HAPPINESS AS PERCEIVED BY PRESENT GENERATION WOMEN

On the basis of many measures the progress of women over recent decades has been extraordinary. The gender wage gap has partly closed and female educational attainment has risen and is now surpassing that of men; women have gained an unprecedented level of control over fertility; technological change in the form of new domestic appliances has freed women from domestic drudgery; and women's freedoms within both the family and market sphere have expanded. Women's lives have become complex: their wellbeing now likely reflects their satisfaction with more facets of life than the women of previous generations. For example, the reported happiness of women who are primarily homemakers might reflect their satisfaction with their home life to a greater extent compared with women who earn their bread and butter and have a family at home. In these latter women, reported happiness may reflect an aggregation of facets over their multiple domains. Social and legal changes have given people more autonomy over individual and family decision making, including rights over marriage, children born out of wedlock and the use of birth control, abortion, and divorce (Stevenson and Wolfers, 2007). During this period there have also been large changes in family life. Divorce rates doubled between the mid-1960s and the mid-1970s, and while they have been falling since the late 1970s, the stock of divorced people has continued to grow (Stevenson and Wolfers, 2007).

Even if women have been made unambiguously better off throughout this period, a richer consideration of the psychology behind happiness might suggest that greater gender equality may lead to a fall in measured well-being. For example, if happiness is assessed relative to outcomes for one's reference group, then greater equality may have led more women to compare their outcomes to those of the men around them. In turn, women might find their relative position lower than when their reference group included only women. This change in the reference group may make women seemingly worse off or it may simply represent a change in their reporting behavior. An alternative form of reference dependent preferences relates well-being to whether or not expectations are met. If the women's movement raised women's expectations faster than society was able to meet them, they are more likely to be disappointed by their actual experienced lives (Kimball and Willis, 2006). As women's expectations move into alignment with their experiences this decline in happiness may reverse. A further alternative suggests that happiness may be driven by good news about lifetime utility (Kimball and Willis, 2006).

There is a blunt disconnect between what most of us think will make us happier and what research shows will actually make us happier. Most of us believe that material or monetary increases will improve our happiness the most (Dunn et al., 2008), whereas a growing body of research shows that the deepest and most stable levels of happiness come from having meaning in our lives (Veenhoven, 2012; Post 2011; Post and Neimark, 2007; Seligman, 2002). But what exactly does it mean to have meanings in our lives? This existential question is examined through the lenses of, in particular, positive psychology research and philosophical induction. It is proposed that individual meaning-making might not be so subjective an exercise as existentialism (human existence as having a set of underlying characteristics, such as anxiety, dread, freedom, awareness of death, and consciousness of existing) generally would suggest. Multidisciplinary research suggests that the major religions might have been right all along with regard to one core message at least: that loving one another generates meaning in our life.

HAPPINESS AND MARRIAGE: MYTH OR REALITY?

Stutzer and Frey (2006) analyzed the causal relationships between marriage and subjective well-being in a longitudinal data set spanning 17 years. They show that happier singles are more likely to opt for marriage and that there are large differences in the benefits from marriage across couples. Potential as well as actual division of labour seems to contribute to spousal well-being, especially for women who all have to raise a young family. In contrast, large differences in the partners' educational levels lead to a negative effect on experienced life satisfaction.

A metanalytic review of nearly 100 studies found marriage to be a strong predictor of life satisfaction, happiness, and overall well-being (Woods et al., 1989). The positive effects of marriage were found to be large. One national survey of 35,000 people in US found that the percentage of married adults who said they were "very happy' (40%) was nearly double that of those who had never been married (26%). Compared to other domains of life (e.g., job status and health), being married and having a family repeatedly show the strongest connection to life satisfaction and happiness (Inglehart et al., 2008).

Subjective well-being research has often found that marriage is positively correlated with well-being. Some have argued that this correlation may be result of happier people being more likely to marry. Others have presented evidence suggesting that the well-being benefits of marriage are short-lasting. A research entitled 'New Evidence on Marriage and the Set Point for Happiness', used data from the British Household Panel Survey (BHPS) to control for individual pre-marital well-being levels or selection effects. Marriage was found to have a positive effect on happiness even after such controls were incorporated. Moreover, new data from the United Kingdom's Annual Population Survey revealed a U-shaped relationship of happiness with age for both married and unmarried people but the dip in happiness in mid-life was found to be more pronounced for unmarried people than for married people, indicating that marriage eases the causes for this dip and its benefits are unlikely to be short-lived. Friendship was considered to be the mechanism through which marriage caused greater life satisfaction. The significance of this mechanism was revealed when it was found that well-being effects of marriage were doubled when a person's spouse was also his/her best friend (Helliwell and Grover, 2014). A study which examined the relationship between interpersonal communications and marital happiness (Juwitaningrum and Basuki, 2006) found it to be significantly positive.

The Implications of "No Strings Attached" for Happiness

A couple walking on the beach holding hands or snuggled up close to each other on a park bench and a single woman enjoying some alone time. Both scenarios are appealing and are potentially associated with high levels of well-being. In today's society decisions to remain single and unattached are respected. Such a decision might be wise even for those who find being in a relationship to be an attractive proposition but learn from experience that they are not comfortable in living up to the commitments that a serious relationship entails. The associated failure in honoring commitments often leads to the termination of relationships with the persons failing then becoming reluctant to enter into new relationships. We now discuss some related researches

An article by Demo and Acock (1996) found that mothers in their first marriage enjoy the highest well-being, mothers in step families fare nearly as well, and divorced and continuously single mothers have the lowest wellbeing. Another study examining wellbeing and choice associated with current marriage trends yielded the following related results: first, unmarried adults attribute being single to both barriers and choices; second, men desire marriage more than women and the never-married want to marry more than the divorced; third, if we categorize both sexes according to whether they are married, divorced or never married then divorced women have the least desire for marriage; fourth, divorced individuals report more life satisfaction than never-married individuals (Frazier et al., 1996).

A study explored single women's views towards the institution of marriage (Perez, 2014). This study utilized a qualitative design with in-depth face-to-face interviews with ten unmarried women living in San Bernardino County being conducted to collect the data. Participants were asked in a structured interview to provide their views in regard to premarital sex, cohabitation, non-marital childbearing, divorce, and same sex marriage. This study found that the extent of conservatism in women's views regarding premarital sex, cohabitation, non-marital childbearing, divorce, and same sex marriage was not impacted by extent of religiosity. The study also found that women commonly held the traditional view that starting a family should be preceded by marriage and the probability of holding such views was not affected by whether premarital sex and cohabitation was accepted by women (Perez, 2014).

A study was conducted to measure life satisfaction among married and unmarried women in India which relied on a sample of 200 women (100 married and 100 unmarried) drawn randomly from the population of Ranchi town. Findings indicated a significantly higher life satisfaction for married women (Ghosh, 2016). On the other hand, a comparison of marital adjustment and subjective wellbeing between samples of 200 each drawn from the populations of Indian educated housewives and married working women revealed significantly higher scores in regard to general health, life satisfaction, and self-esteem measures and lower scores in regard to hopelessness, insecurity, and anxiety for the latter group. This leads us to the conclusion that working women did significantly better in terms of both marital adjustment and wellbeing which in turn indicates the salutary impact of a working life outside home on mental health (Nathawat and Mathur, 1993). Housewives though had lower scores on negative affect than working women.

Love and Happiness: Do the Two Go Hand-in-Hand?

When one is unhappily single, it is easy to assume that love would remedy the lack of happiness. But does it? Researchers have long tried to determine if there is a correlation between happiness and the thing we call 'love'. The hypothesis that single young adults who perceive their singlehood as voluntary would report a higher level of positive mental health (i.e., emotional, psychological and social well-being) and lower levels of mental illness (i.e., somatic symptoms, anxiety, social dysfunction, severe depression etc.) and romantic loneliness than young adults who perceive their singlehood as involuntary was tested (Adamczyk, 2016). This paper also investigated whether it is romantic loneliness which accounts for the difference in the levels of positive mental health and mental illness experienced, if any, by those who are voluntarily and involuntarily single. Quite expectedly, voluntarily single young adults reported a lower level of romantic loneliness than involuntarily single young adults, but the two groups did not differ in regard to either the extent of positive mental health or the incidence of mental health problems. In addition, gender differences were observed solely in the domain of romantic loneliness, with women reporting greater romantic loneliness than men. The mediation analysis revealed that romantic loneliness did not affect the extent of positive mental health and the incidence of mental illness unequally across the two groups of voluntarily single and involuntarily single adults with both voluntary and involuntary singlehood being predictive of somatic symptoms, anxiety and insomnia, severe depression, and romantic loneliness.

When the relationships among psychopathy, romantic relationships, and wellbeing were investigated in 431 undergraduates, it was seen that for both males and females, various components of romantic relationship quality were positively correlated with subjective well-being (SWB) and negatively correlated with ill-being. However, only for females was overall romantic relationship quality positively correlated with life satisfaction, happiness, and positive affect, and negatively correlated with negative affect and depression (Love and Holder, 2015).

According to Markey et al. (2007) the perception of happy kinship is associated with relationship quality and actual good health. The participants in their study perceived their romantic partners to be primarily positive health influences; women believed their partners were more influential than did men and eating and physical activity were believed to be most affected by partners. A direct association was revealed between relationship quality and health of participants on the one hand and reports of the perceived health influences of partners on the other.

Gere and Schimmack (2013) found that goal conflict, as reported by a partner, adversely impacted relationship quality and this effect was manifested in lower subjective wellbeing of the other partner. A general observation which emerged was that lower relationship quality was inevitably associated with lower subjective happiness.

A study aimed to see the difference in loneliness between a middle-aged unmarried woman and a married associate (Rakhmiatie and Widyarini, 2006). The answer that emerged was that the first type of adult experienced more social and emotional loneliness than the second type of adult, with the first type of loneliness impacting the subject when she was alone and sometimes even in a crowd.

One Can Be Happy Being Alone

While many people think of their marriages as a source of happiness it is possible for a single adult also to be happy. A study of 24,000 people in Germany over 15 years by Tara Parker-Pope, revealed that getting married only triggered a small bump in happiness, measured as one-tenth of a point on an 11- point scale. Of course, there were big variations among individuals. Some people were much happier after marriage; however, sadly, some reported less happiness after marriage. The bottom line was that if someone is already happy, she/he will not gain much extra happiness from marriage which will not have a significant impact on a social network that is already rich and is the cause of high pre-marital happiness. The extra companionship of marriage, while nice, doesn't have a marked impact on her/his overall sense of happiness. At the same time, if someone lacks a strong social network, she/he would get a bigger happiness benefit from partnering up. At the same time, a married person with a limited social network will suffer more after divorce or the death of a spouse.

In summary:

1. Individual personality tends to influence overall happiness irrespective of whether a person is married.
2. Happier people are more likely to get married.
3. Marriage triggers a short bump in happiness, but after two years, everyone settles back and stagnates to one level.
4. Improving our social connections and relationships is good for overall happiness. But if one is not married, or does not have a happy marriage, one can still improve her/his happiness by nurturing their friendships and social connections.

CONCLUSION

Thus, to sum matters up it can be said that happiness can be explained by a variety of factors: life satisfaction, appreciation of life, moments of pleasure etc. But at a tautological level happiness results from the experiencing of positive emotions. Through an extensive literature review and a primary survey this paper establishes that such positive emotional experiences and therefore happiness can result from close relationships among humans. That is, other things remaining the same, those involved in close relationships, based on mutual disclosure and emotional bonding, are happier than others.

The science of close relationships boils down to fundamental lessons that are obvious and difficult to master: empathy, positivity and a strong emotional connection drive the happiest and healthiest relationships. However, yet some people are not happy enough for the fact that they often fail to see the brighter aspects of events and difficult situations. Remaining single with simply being in love with self can be equally satisfying. The process of learning to master happiness is indeed a journey towards enlightenment.

REFERENCES

Adamczyk, K. (2016). Voluntary and Involuntary single-hood and young adults' mental health: An investigation of mediating role of romantic loveliness. *Current Psychology*, 36(4): 888–904.

Albuquerque, I., Lima, M., Matos, M. and Figueiredo, C. (2013). The interplay among levels of personality: The mediator effect of personal projects between the big five and subjective well-being. *Journal of Happiness Studies*, 14(1): 235–250.

Alexander, M., Garda, L., Kanade, S., Jejecbhoy, S. and Ganatra, B. (2007). Correlates of premarital relationships among unmarried youth in Pune district, Maharashtra, India. *International Family Planning Perspective*, 33(4): 150-159.

Andrade, A.L.D., Wachelke, J.F.R., Beatriz, A. and Rodrigues, C.H. (2015). Relationship satisfaction in young adults. *Gender and Love Dimensions*, 9 (1): 19–31.

Cheng, H., and Furnham, A. (2001). Attributional style and personality as predictor of happiness and mental health. *Journal of Happiness Studies*, 2(3): 307–327.

Demo, D.H. and Acock, A.C. (1996). Single hood, marriage, and remarriage: The effects of family structure and family relationships on mothers' well-being. *Journal of Family Issues*, 17(3): 388–407.

Diener, R. (2009). The magic of love. *PsycCRITIQUES*, 54(32).

Frazier, P., Arikian, N., Benson, S., Losoff, A. and Maurer, S. (1006). Desire for marriage and life satisfaction among unmarried heterosexual adults. *Journal of Social and Personal Relationships*, 13(2): 225–239.

Gere, J. and Schimmack, U. (2013). When romantic partners' goals conflict: Effects on relationship quality and subjective well-being. *Journal of Happiness Studies*, 14 (1): 37–49.

Ghosh, S.M. (2016). Life satisfaction among married and unmarried women of Ranchi Town. *International Journal of Scientific Research*, Vol. 5 (4).

Helliwell, J.F. and Grover, S. (2014). How's life at home? New evidence on marriage and the set point for happiness. NBER Working Paper No. 20794. NBER Program(s).

Helliwell, J.F., Layard, R., and Sachs, J. (2019). *World Happiness Report 2019.* New York: Sustainable Development Solutions Network.

Inglehart, R., Foa, R., Peterson, C. and Welzel, C. (2008). Development, freedom, and rising happiness: A global perspective. *Perspectives on Psychological Science*, 3: 264–285.

Juwitaningrum, Y. and Basuki, A.M.H. (2006). Relationship Between Interpersonal Communication with Happiness. In Marriage Husband Wife Partner. Undergraduate Program.

Kimball, M. and Willis, R. (2006). Utility and happiness. University of Michigan. mimeo.

Lauriola, M. and Iani, L. (2017). Personality, positivity, and happiness: A mediation analysis using a bifactor model. *Journal of Happiness Studies*, 18: 1659–1682.

Love, A.B. and Holder, M.D. (2016). Can romantic relationship quality mediate the relation between psychopathy and subjective well-being? *Journal of Happiness Studies*, 17: 2407–2429.

Lu, L. and Hu, C.H. (2005). Personality leisure experiences and happiness. *Journal of Happiness Studies*, 6(3): 325–342.

Lyubomirsky, S. (2008). *The How of Happiness: A New Approach to getting the life you want.* New York, NY: Penguin Books.

Lyubomirsky, S., Sheldon K.M. and Schkade, D. (2005). Pursuing happiness: The architecture of sustainable change. *Review of General Psychology*, 9: 111–131.

Markey, C.N., Markey, P.M. and Gray, H.F. (2007). Romantic relationships and health: An examination of individuals' perceptions of their romantic partners' influences on their health. *Sex Roles*, 57.

McMahon, D. (2006). *Happiness: A History. New York*, NY: Atlantic Monthly Press.

Nathawat, S.S. and Mathur, A. (1993). Marital adjustment and subjective well-being in Indian educated housewives and working women. *The Journal of Psychology—Interdisciplinary and Applied*, 127 (3).

Perez, Y. (2014). *Single women's views toward the institution of Marriage.* Electronic theses, Projects, Dissertations. Paper 79.

Pollock, N.C., Noser, A.E., Holden, C.J. and Hill, V.Z. (2016). Do orientations to happiness mediate the association bet, personality traits and subjective wellbeing? *Journal of Happiness Studies*, 17(2): 713–729.

Post, S. and Neimark, J. (2007). *Why good things happen to good people: The exciting new research that provides the link between doing good and living a longer, healthier, happier life.* New York: Broadway Books.

Seligman, M.E.P. (2002). *Authentic happiness: Using the new positive psychology to realize your potential for lasting fulfillment.* New York: Free Press.

Sternberg, R.J. (2007). Triangulating Love. In Oord, T.J. *The Altruism Reader: Selections from Writings on Love, Religion, and Science.* West Conshohocken, PA: Templeton Foundation. p. 332. ISBN 9781599471273, 2007.

Stevenson Driving Forces. *Journal of Economic Perspectives*, 21(2): 27–52.

Stutzer, A. and Frey, B.S. (2006). Does marriage make people happy, or do happy people get married? *Journal of Socio-Economics* 35(2): 326–347.

Tara Parker-Pope; author of *"For Better: The Science of a Good Marriage."* Illustrations by Esther Aarts.

Veenhoven, R. (2010). Greater happiness for a greater number – is that possible and desirable? *Journal of Happiness Studies*, 11(5): 605–629.

Warner, R. and Vroman, K. (2011). Happiness inducing behaviors in everyday life: An, B. and Wolfers, J. (2007). Marriage and Divorce: Changes and Their empirical assessment of 'the how of happiness. *Journal of Happiness Studies*, 12(6):1063–1082.

Wood, W., Rhodes, N. and Whelan, M. (1989). Sex differences in positive well-being: A consideration of emotional style and marital status. *Psychological Bulletin*, 106(2): 249–264.

In: A Socio-Economic and Demographic ... ISBN: 978-1-53619-023-6
Editors: A. Rodriguez Andres et al. © 2021 Nova Science Publishers, Inc.

Chapter 6

MENTAL HEALTH SCENARIO IN INDIA

*Abhay Kumar De**

Consultant, Department of Psychiatry,
Ramakrishna Mission Seva Pratisthan Hospital and Vivekananda
Institute of Medical Sciences, Kolkata, India

ABSTRACT

India is plagued by a severe mental health problem: roughly one out of seven Indians affected by mental disorders and a suicide mortality rate as high as 16 per 100,000. The government has responded very well through a national mental health policy, a rights-based mental health act and a mental health program which attempts to link service at the doorstep of every household to the network of primary and community health centres, mental hospitals and nodal centres. Yet major problems remain, primarily those arising from paucity of skilled manpower such as psychiatrists, clinical psychologists, and mental health care workers; and the long distances often separating the household and quality medical care. The government should thus give top priority to programs for infrastructure creation and human capital formation in regard to mental health care. Prevention of mental illness and promotion of mental health

---

* Corresponding Author's E-mail: drabhaydey@rediffmail.com.

needs to be integrated within a public policy approach that encompasses horizontal action through different public sectors such as environment, housing, social welfare, labor and employment, education, criminal justice, and human rights. This will generate wide ranging health, social and economic benefits.

Keywords: mental health, suicide rates, health care

INTRODUCTION

India, the ancient land of Pranayama, Yoga, Vipassana meditation, and other wonderful treasures, with focus on simple living and lofty thinking leading to physical and mental well-being, has given much riches to Oriental and Occidental thought. Its sages and philosophers have contributed immensely to the advancement of science and also beamed light towards the path of mental enlightenment. A note on the mentioned techniques for promoting mental wellbeing is in order. Vipassana is a technique of meditation which is an observation-based, self-exploratory journey that focuses on the deep interconnection between the mind and body. The goal is to create awareness of the deep mind or deep consciousness. Pranayama is the practice of breath control in Yoga which helps in harmonising the body systems. Yoga is essentially a spiritual discipline based on an extremely subtle science, which focuses on bringing harmony between the mind and the body. Yogic practices and meditation techniques, especially mindfulness techniques, are being extensively utilized in modern medicine – for example, in the branches of psychiatry or mental health, cardio-vascular and chest medicine and so on.

However, when we reflect on the current status of mental health in India, the picture is far from rosy. The benefits of the richness of Indian thought and mental enlightenment of the Rishis have not permeated down to the grassroots level. The figures capturing the extent of mental illnesses in India from the National Mental Health Survey of India, an extensive meticulous survey of 39532 individuals, conducted by NIMHANS (National Institute of Mental Health and Neuro-Sciences), Bangalore, paint a not so rosy picture. Another recent extensive study, 'The burden of mental disorders across the states of India: The Global Burden of Disease Study, 1990-2017', also throws up a similar far from encouraging picture of the mental health scenario in India (Sagar et al., 2020).

According to World Health Organisation (WHO, 2004): "Mental health is a state of wellbeing in which an individual realizes his or her own abilities, can cope with the normal stresses of life, can work productively and fruitfully, and is able to make a contribution to his or her community." It may be noted that the positive dimension of mental health is stressed in the 1948 WHO definition of health (as contained in its Constitution) – "A state of complete physical, mental and social well-being and not merely absence of disease or infirmity."

The figures capturing the extent of mental health problems in India are staggering and humbling. As per the National Mental Health Survey (NMHS) of India, the estimated current prevalence of mental morbidity in individuals above 18 years (excluding tobacco use disorders) is 10.6% and lifetime prevalence, the proportion of population that has experienced mental morbidity at least once in its life, is 13.7%. According to NMHS, depression affects 1 in 20 people during their lifetime, while nearly 22% of the population suffers from substance use disorders (use of addicting agents) during lifetime and 1.9% are affected with severe mental disorders (SMDs). Children and adolescents are one of the most severely affected age groups, and suicide is emerging as a major concern with 1% population reported to have a high suicide risk. According to the WHO Mental Health Atlas of 2017 the suicide mortality rate in India is 16.3 per 100,000 persons.

According to NMHS about 150 million Indians or more than 10% of the population are in need of active interventions. It found that the weighted prevalence, the sum of the products of illness specific prevalence and attached weight where weights capture the severity of the mental illness, across diagnostic categories was higher in urban metros than in rural and urban non-metro areas (those urban agglomerations with less than 10 million populations each). However, differences existed across diagnostic categories. The prevalence of schizophrenia and other psychoses (0.64%), mood disorders (5.6%) and neurotic and stress related disorders (6.93%) in the urban metros was about 2-3 times that in urban non-metro areas and rural areas. The authors of the mentioned report opined that the higher prevalence could be attributed to several factors such as fast-paced lifestyle, stress, complexities of living, breakdown of support systems and challenges posed by economic instability. However, further studies are needed to understand the relationship between urbanisation and mental illness. With continued urbanisation the burden is expected to rise and hence, there is a need for an urban specific mental health programme.

According to the mentioned Global Burden of Disease (GBD) Study, 1990-2017, which was carried out for the various states of India, one in seven Indians is affected by mental disorders. The high burden of mental and substance use disorders can be attributed to the significant incidence of severe mental disorders (SMDs), which include Schizophrenia, Bipolar disorder, Major Depressive Disorder and other psychotic disorders. There is also a significant contribution from Common mental disorders (CMDs) which include anxiety disorders, depression, somatoform and other neurotic disorders and substance abuse disorders. According to this study, in the year 2017 there were an estimated 197.3 million people with mental illness in India, including 45.7 million with depressive disorder, and 44.9 million with anxiety disorder. Thus, 14.7% of the Indian population was suffering from mental illness.

The significance of any disabling illness can be measured through the number of Disability Adjusted Life Years (DALYs) attributable to this illness. The use of the concept of DALYs is becoming increasingly popular in the field of Public Health and Health Impact Assessment (HIA) and is prominent in the mentioned GBD study. DALYs not only include years of life lost due to premature death, but also equivalent years of 'healthy' life lost by virtue of being in states of poor health and disability. In so doing morbidity (sickness) and mortality (death) are combined into a single metric. The GBD study points out that the contribution of mental disorders to the total DALYs in India increased from 2.5% in 1990 to 4.7% in 2017; thus, the proportional contribution of mental disorders to the total disease burden in India has almost doubled since 1990. Depressive disorders contributed the most to the total DALYs attributed to mental disorders (33.8%) followed by anxiety disorders (19.0%), Idiopathic Developmental Intellectual Disability (10.8%), Schizophrenia (9.8%), Bipolar disorder (6.9%), Conduct disorder (5.9%), Autism spectrum disorder (3.2%), Eating disorder (2.2%) and Attention deficit hyperactivity disorder (0.3%). All other mental disorders comprised 8.0% of these DALYs. Furthermore, a significant correlation between the prevalence of depressive disorder and the incidence of death due to suicides was found at the state level for females and males. What is very alarming is that the suicide rate among Indian females was double the global suicide death rate (Dandona et al., 2018).

Mental and substance use disorders (use of various addicting agents) create a huge burden on the patients, their families and society [6-9]. Most mental disorders have onset at a young age and last a long time affecting the most productive years of life. The illness affects almost all aspects of life including personal, familial, occupational and social areas. Added to this is the stigma and discrimination in society which can manifest as difficulty in getting a job and retaining it. This makes the persons with mental illness unable to function at their full potential. Not just the patients themselves, but even their families face problems as they have to spend a lot of time and money in their role as main caregivers in the absence of state support. This affects the caregivers' own functioning in different areas. They face financial problems due to the high cost of treatment and also have to take breaks from their jobs (Ganguly et al., 2010).

DeHert et al. (2010) have pointed out that persons with mental illness are prone to developing different medical problems such as nutritional deficiencies, cardiovascular and metabolic disorders, and infectious disease, further adding to the burden. There is also tremendous loss of productive years. The life span of the patients with schizophrenia, bipolar disorder, and depression and substance use disorders is often shortened due to the associated severe physical problems and deaths due to accidents and suicide. Early intervention is required to prevent mental illness and promote good mental health. Importantly, the positive association of depressive disorders and schizophrenia with suicide deaths in India implies that attention through primary care to these illnesses is urgently needed for suicide prevention. Special attention should be given to females because, as mentioned previously, Indian women have double the global suicide death rate.

When we look at the situation globally to compare it to the Indian situation, it is found that even in wealthy countries, 40-60% of people with severe mental disorders do not receive the care they need. Murthi (2016), writing in the Indian Journal of Social Psychiatry (IJSP) about the mental health situation in the world, quoted a review article where it is stated that "when it comes to mental health, all countries are developing countries". The World Health Organization (WHO) reported in 2001 that 450 million people worldwide suffered from some form of mental disorder or brain condition. The 'Global Burden of Disease Study' by the Institute of Health Metrics and Evaluation by Ritchie et al. comes up with an estimate of 972 million, which is 12.94% of the world population of 7511 million, for this variable in 2017. The figure of 12.94% is quite close to 14.73%, the figure estimated by the GBD study.

Interestingly, according to a World Health Organization Global Study by Demyttenaere, et al. (2004) the United States, Colombia, the Netherlands, and Ukraine tend to have high prevalence estimates across most classes of mental disorders, while places such as Nigeria, Shanghai and Italy have lower prevalence. Prevalence was also lower in the Asian countries in general. Nevertheless, the figures from developing countries may be underestimates because of lack of proper reporting and also because they may be overburdened with other problems such as poverty, war and other illnesses including infectious diseases. According to Ritchie and Roser (2020) – "Diagnosis statistics alone would not bring us close to the true figure — mental health is typically under-reported, and under-diagnosed. If relying on mental health diagnoses alone, prevalence figures would be likely to reflect healthcare spending (which allows for more focus on mental health disorders) rather than giving a representative perspective on differences between countries; high-income countries would likely show significantly higher prevalence as a result of more diagnoses."

A prominent message from a WHO publication on Social Determinants of Mental Health, 2017, is that action and public policies to address existing health inequalities need to be universal and inclusive, yet proportionate to need. Targeting resources at the most disadvantaged groups alone runs the risk of detracting from the overall goal of reducing the steepness of the social gradient in health. The authors also state that since risk and protective factors for mental health act at different levels, responses to them need to be multi-layered and multi-sectoral. Health, education, welfare, transport, and housing sectors all need to be concerned and involved, and contribute to a 'health in all policies' approach. Certain population subgroups are at higher risk of mental disorders because of greater exposure and vulnerability to unfavorable social, economic and environmental circumstances, interrelated with gender. Disadvantage starts before birth and accumulates throughout life. A significant body of work now exists that emphasizes the need for a life-course approach to understanding and tackling mental and physical health inequalities. This approach accounts for the differential experience and impact of social determinants throughout life. A life-course approach proposes actions to improve the condition in which people are born and grow, live, work and age. Actions that prevent mental disorders and promote mental health are an essential part of efforts to improve the health of the world's population and to reduce health inequalities. There is firm consensus on known protective and risk factors for mental disorders. In addition, a growing body of evidence exists, not only from high-income countries, but also from low and middle-income countries, that shows effective actions can be successfully implemented at all stages of development. A key concept proposed is proportionate universalism, i.e. policies should be universal yet proportionate to need. Focusing solely on the most disadvantaged people will fail to achieve the required reduction in health inequalities necessary to reduce the steepness of the social gradient in health. Therefore, it is important that actions be universal yet calibrated proportionately to the level of disadvantage.

Risk and protective factors act at several different levels, including the family, the community, the structural and the population levels. A 'social determinants of health approach' requires action across multiple sectors and levels. Taking a life course perspective recognizes that influences that operate at each stage of life can affect mental health. Social arrangements and institutions such as education, social care and work have a huge impact on the opportunities that empower people to choose their own course in life. Experience with these social arrangements and institutions differs enormously and their structures and impacts are, to a greater or lesser extent, influenced or mitigated by national and transnational policies. Good mental health is integral to human health and well-being. A person's mental health and the incidence of many common mental disorders is shaped by various social, economic, and physical environments operating at different stages of life. Risk factors for many common mental disorders are strongly associated with social inequalities: the greater the social inequality the higher the inequality in risk. The authors of the WHO publication, *Social Determinants of Mental Health* opined that it is of major importance that action is taken to improve the conditions of everyday life, beginning before birth and progressing into early childhood and adolescence, during family building and working ages, and through to old age. Action throughout these life stages would provide opportunities for both improving population mental health (the overall mental health status of the people at large), and for reducing risk of being affected with those mental disorders that are associated with social inequalities. Where comprehensive action across the life course is needed, there is considerable evidence and scientific consensus that action to give every child the best possible start in life will generate the greatest societal and mental health benefits. In order to achieve this, action needs to be universal, across the whole of the social distribution, and it should be proportionate to disadvantage in order to level the social gradient and successfully reduce inequalities in mental disorders.

The global burden due to mental and neurological disorders increased from 10.5% of total DALYs in 1990 to 14% in 2005 (see Murray and Lopez, 1996; Deds et al., 2001; WHO report; and Prince et al., 2007)

According to a WH0 estimate, 7.4% of global DALYs were caused by mental behavioural disorders alone. Depression, bipolar disorder, schizophrenia, alcohol and substance use disorders are the major contributors to Global Burden of Disease (GBD) due to neuropsychiatric disorders. Murray et al. (2012) opined that burden caused by mental disorders is estimated to be higher than that due to HIV/AIDS, tuberculosis, diabetes, urogenital, blood and endocrine disorders. In 2010 it was estimated that in 20 years, the global effect of mental disorders in terms of lost economic output would be to the extent of US $16 trillion (Bloom et al., 2011). In 2015 substance use disorders were ranked as the fifth leading cause of DALYs and the estimated global prevalence of depressive and anxiety disorders was 253 million and 266 million respectively (as per the Global Burden of Disease Study).

In what follows we first take a look at global developments to tackle the problem of mental health in Section 2 and then examine how these developments have found a resonance in mental health programmes, policies, development of infrastructure and innovation in India.

GLOBAL EFFORTS TO ADDRESS THE MENTAL HEALTH PROBLEM

The world community is gradually waking up to the grim reality of the problem of mental health and its far-reaching implications as is evidenced by the following (mentioning only a few): (i) 2004 WHO report - Prevention of mental disorders; (ii) 2008 European Union Pact for mental disorders (iii) 2011 US national prevention strategy which aimed to guide the country most effectively towards health and wellbeing; and (iv) 2011 UK strategy paper – "No health without mental health". In 2016 there were two significant developments. First, the World Bank endorsed mental health as a global development priority. Second, mental health was explicitly included in the Sustainable Development Goals, the UN development agenda that will guide global and national agendas for the next 15 years. These developments have created a unique opportunity to work across sectors to optimise health funding, research, and capacity building programmes.

Four major reasons have been identified by various authors as to why a majority of people across the globe needing mental health care do not receive it: a) stigma; b) human resource shortage; c) fragmented service delivery; and d) lack of research capacity (for implementation of policy change).

Stigma is very commonly associated with mental illnesses. Stigma occurs when society labels someone as tainted or less desirable. Stigma in this case consists of three elements: a lack of knowledge (ignorance) about mental illnesses, negative attitudes (prejudice) and people behaving in ways that disadvantage the stigmatized person (discrimination). Stigma can also be seen in the current world towards Covid 19 patients. Two major types of stigma associated with mental health problems are social stigma and self-stigma. Social stigma, also called public stigma, refers to negative stereotypes in society of those with mental illnesses. Self-stigma occurs when a person internalises negative stereotypes. This can lead to low self-esteem, shame and hopelessness. Stigma can hinder mental health treatment and recovery and also hamper detection as people may be reluctant to disclose mental illness.

Human resource shortage is a problem observed all over the world. There is gross lack of trained manpower to attend to the needs of mentally ill patients. Resources are fragmented and concentrated mainly in urban areas. Research has focused more on infectious diseases and non-communicable diseases such as cardiovascular disease, diabetes and cancers. Mental illnesses have usually been accorded low priority in the allocation of funds for research.

Experts have stressed that the pursuit of the following objectives should be given priority and focused attention: (i) diminishing pervasive stigma; (ii) building a system for mental health treatment and research capacity; (iii) implementing prevention programmes to decrease incidence of mental disorders and (iv) establishing sustainable scale -up of the public health systems.

Stigma can only be reduced by creating mass awareness that mental illnesses are brain disorders and treatable like other illnesses affecting the human body. This needs concerted efforts by the government and also non-government players using mass media and other channels complemented by an increase in the level of education of the population.

Prevention programmes to decrease the incidence of mental illnesses needs a life-course approach to improve the overall health of the population as stated previously. The concept of positive mental health is also coming into vogue.

Some WHO core programmes undertaken to meet the challenges may be cited as below:

1. WHO MIND (Mental Health In Development)

This project works to unite and empower people to improve service delivery and human rights conditions in mental health facilities and social care homes. It is part of WHO's Quality Rights campaign to end violations against people with mental disabilities.

2. Mental Health Gap Action Programme (The mhGAP Programme):

The treatment gap (difference between number of persons needing treatment and those who actually get it as a proportion of the former figure) is huge. It is estimated to be between 76-85% for low and middle-income countries (LMICS) and 35-50% for high income countries (HICs). This programme aims to bridge this gap.

In 2011 WHO estimated a minimum shortage of 1.18 million health professionals including 55000 Psychiatrists, 628320 nurses in mental health settings and 493000 psycho-social care providers worldwide.

A new concept has emerged to meet the needs of manpower - 'task sharing' (initially called task shifting). This consists of transferring clinical duties to trained lay health workers. This will help a large extent to offset the shortage of doctors and other trained personnel.

3. GCPN (Global Clinical Practise Network)

Created by WHO's department of mental health and substance abuse, it holds promise for promoting collaborative initiatives that enhance training, research and clinical capacity for dealing with mental health issues worldwide.

It represents an important part of WHO's efforts to make isolated research silos a thing of the past and bring evidence based mental health care to those who need it most (especially LMICS), thereby reducing the gap between research and clinical implementation.

It comprises straightforward and specific user-friendly guidelines for diagnosing mental illnesses and providing evidence-based practices (EBPS) for better treatment. This can improve the quality of mental health care worldwide.

In this regard, mention must be made of the Comprehensive Mental Health Action Plan for 2013-20. It was adopted by the 66th World Health Assembly in 2013. According to this plan all United Nations members states are committed to providing mental health care that is integrated into primary health care and subsumes both common and severe mental disorders.

Four major objectives were set forth: strengthening of effective leadership and governance for mental health; provision of comprehensive, integrated and responsive mental health and social care services in community-based settings; implementation of strategies for promotion and prevention in mental health; and strengthening information systems, evidence and research for mental health.

Tackling the Mental Health Problem in India: Programmes, Infrastructure and Innovations

It may be noted that India was one of the first developing countries to recognise the need to address the problem of mental health. This was done through the National Mental Health Programme (NMHP) launched in 1982 by the Government of India. Subsequently, The National Mental Health Policy was introduced in 2014 and a rights based Mental Healthcare Act in 2017 which replaced the Mental Healthcare Act of 1987.The child health programme under the National Health Mission and the National Adolescent Health Programme includes components to address the mental health of children and adolescents. These are significant measures, especially if we consider that the WHO, in a report in 2001, reported the absence of a mental health policy in more than 40% of countries and of a mental health legislation in around 25% of countries.

The main objectives of NMHP were to a) ensure the availability and accessibility of minimal mental health care for all in the foreseeable future; b) encourage the application of mental health knowledge in general health care and in social development; c) promote community participation in mental health service development; and d) enhance human resources in mental health sub-specialties. NMHP was re-launched as the District Mental Health Programme (DMHP) in 1996. The programme was re-strategized in 2003 to include two schemes viz. modernisation of state mental hospitals and up-gradation of psychiatry wings of Medical colleges/General Hospitals. In 2009 a man power development scheme became part of this programme and involved creation of centres of excellence and the setting up of post graduate departments of mental health facilities in an effort to impart training and expertise to meet the needs of adequately trained manpower.

Currently we are in the 12th Plan Period and the DMHP stands at the threshold of reaching its potential in considerable measure to ultimately realize the goals set for it at the outset. The main objective of the DMHP is to provide community mental health services and facilitate integration of mental health with general health services through decentralisation of treatment from specialised mental hospital-based care to primary health care services. On the basis of the 'Bellary model' (a pilot project undertaken in Bellary district of Karnataka), the DMHP was launched in 1996 in four districts under NMHP. It was expanded to 27 districts of the country by the end of the 1X Th Five Year Plan period. As of now, 241 districts are under the DMHP under the X11th 5-year plan. It is proposed to expand the DMHP to all districts in a phased manner.

The DMHP envisages a community based approach to the issue of mental health which includes the provision of mental out-patient and in-patient services; an outreach component consisting of satellite clinics operating in Community Health Centres (CHCs)/ Primary Health Centres (PHCs) as well as life - skill education and counselling in schools, college counselling services, counselling for stress management at the workplace, and suicide prevention services; and sensitisation and training of health personnel at the district and sub-district levels. This programme would also include camps for generation of awareness about mental illness and related stigma which would involve local PRIs (Panchayati Raj Institutions), faith healers, teachers, leaders etc. It would also involve community participation facilitated through linkages with self-help groups, family and caregiver groups and NGOs (Non-Government Organisations) working in the field of mental health, and sensitisation of enforcement officials regarding legal provisions for effective implementation of Mental Health Act.

The DMHP would involve hiring of various kinds of manpower on contractual basis: psychiatrist, clinical psychologist, psychiatric nurse, psychiatric social worker, community nurse, monitoring and evaluation officer, case registry assistant, and ward assistant/orderly. An annual financial support of Rs 8.32 million per DMHP unit has been envisioned.

Evaluation has revealed that the DMHP is working to an extent but there are certain shortcomings. One is the long distance of the outreach camps from the nodal centres. This is causing the healthcare staff to lose valuable time in transit. Second, active treatment of mental patients by doctors at the primary health care level is not observed frequently because of various reasons: the large burden of patients suffering from other illnesses; doctors not being confident enough to treat mentally ill patients after only a short 3-day training; the Mental Health Care Act (MHCA), 2017 allowing only treatment for 72 hours by a physician before referral to a higher centre; and other legal issues. Thus, the whole exercise is probably not bearing the desired results (as opined in Singh, 2019; Sagar et al., 2017 and Chakraborty, 2018.)

Thus, in spite of efforts by the government, the provision of mental health services in India has been poor as revealed by a high treatment gap for mental disorders, poor evidence-based treatment, and gender-differentials in treatment (according to Sagar et al., 2017; Grover et al., 2019; Petersen et al., 2017; Mugisha et al., 2017; Sidhaye et al., 2015; Kaur et al., 2017; Arvind et al., 2019). The suicide mortality rate per 100,000 populations is 16.3 (WHO Mental Health Atlas, 2017). India's total healthcare spending (out-of-pocket and public) is approximately 3.6% of GDP according to OECD (Organisation for Economic Cooperation and Development) and 3.53% according to World Bank and WHO data in 2017. These figures compare poorly with many countries. The total health expenditure by the Centre and the states for financial year 2019-20 was 2.6 trillion Rupees or 1.29 % of GDP of which a mere 1.3% was spent on mental health (WHO Atlas, 2017).

As per the WHO Mental Health Atlas of 2017, mental health resources in India consist of 1.93 mental health workers per 100000 persons including 0.29 psychiatrists, 0.80 mental health nurses, 0.07 psychologists, 0.06 social workers, 0.03 occupational therapists, 0.17 speech therapists and 0.36 other paid mental health workers. The numbers are grossly inadequate, as noted by various experts. The state wise availability of psychiatrists (per 100,000 persons) varies from 0.05 in Madhya Pradesh to 1.2 in Kerala. Except for Kerala, all other states are short of the minimum requirement of at least 1 psychiatrist per 100,000 persons. Kerala also has the highest number of clinical psychologists per 100,000 persons (0.6) in India as noted by Srinivasa (2017).

Keeping the above inadequacy in healthcare manpower in mind, steps are being taken to boost the supply line by increasing training facilities.

There are approximately 133 medical colleges and post graduate institutes in India which admit around 327 students for MD Degree in Psychiatry (Doctor of Psychological Medicine) each year, besides which 56 medical colleges have training facilities for 125 DPM (Diploma in Psychological Medicine) students. In addition, 50-60 post graduates appear every year for exam leading to the award of DNB (Diplomate of National Board) in psychiatry, as noted by Awasthi et al. (2015). The focus has been on an increase in the training facilities in psychiatry, clinical psychology, psychiatric social work and psychiatry nursing in the newly established centres of excellence under the National Mental Health Programme (NMHP) in India. But still the required numbers will be difficult to achieve in near future as stated by Murthy (2011).

To increase the number of qualified mental health professionals in the country, the government is implementing manpower development schemes for the establishment of Centres of Excellence and strengthening /establishment of Post Graduate (PG) Departments in mental health institutions under the NMHP.

Coming to infrastructure, a total of 952 mental health outpatient facilities attached to hospitals exist in India. There are 1217 'community based /non-hospital' mental health out-patient facilities and 240 other outpatient facilities (e.g., mental health day care or treatment facility). There are 139 outpatient facilities specifically for children and adolescents (including services for developmental disorders) and 67 other outpatient services for children and adolescents (e.g., day care). In-patient services are available at 136 mental hospitals, 389 psychiatric units in general hospitals, 15 forensic in-patient units and 223 residential care facilities. There are 45 in-patient facilities specifically for children and adolescents. These numbers are, however, inadequate considering the vast population of about 1400 million (WHO Atlas, 2017).

Let us come specifically to the situation in rural India. Some authors like Kumar (2011), Meltzer (2008), and Thara et al. (2004) have noted a silence on mental health services in rural India in the National Rural Health Mission (NRHM), and observed that there has been little effort to improve the rural mental health services Chatterjee (2009) and Pathare (2011) point out that this is a matter of serious concern in view of increased population, changing values and life-style, frequent disruption in income due to crop failures, natural calamities like drought and floods, economic crisis, unemployment, lack of social support and increasing insecurity – all of these factors or phenomena are expected to contribute to a substantial increase in the number of people suffering from mental illness in rural areas. A 2005 report by the National Commission on Macroeconomics and Health (NCMH) shows that at least 6.5% of the Indian population suffers from some form of serious mental disorders with no discernible rural-urban difference in incidence. As 72.2% of the Indian population live in rural areas with only about 25% of the health infrastructure, medical manpower and other health resources, it may be surmised that the number of people affected with any mental and behavioural disorder but lacking treatment might be high in rural areas as pointed out by Kumar (2011) and Gururaj et al. (2005).

Despite NRHM initiatives, general health services in rural areas are not adequate and struggling because of deficiency in infrastructure and human resources and other problems. Rural areas account for 31.9% of all government hospital beds and given that rural population is in excess of 70% of the total population, the current bed-population ratio of 1.1 bed per 1000 in urban areas is more than 5 times the rural ratio of 0.2 as per figures derived from National Commission on Macroeconomics and Health Background Papers, 2005. In regard to rural areas, the numbers of doctors in primary health centres (PHC), specialists at community health centres (CHC), male health workers and female health workers reveal shortages of 8%, 65%, 55.3% and 12.6% respectively (Ministry of Health & Family Welfare, GOI, 2007 Bulletin on rural health statistics). On the whole rural India has access to just 0.2 psychiatrists, 0.05 psychiatric nurses, 0.03 psychologists per 100,000 persons; and 0.26 mental health beds – 0.2 in mental hospitals and 0.05 in general hospitals – per 10000 persons (WHO Mental Health Atlas, 2015). Thus, access is very low. Around 2011, it was estimated that India needed about 140000 psychiatrists as opposed to the existing figure of 3000 out of which 75% worked in urban areas with less than 28% of the population (WHO, 2001).

Given the limited or no service availability, the treatment gap is huge in rural areas. Barriers to seeking help in rural areas are many: unavailability of mental health services, low literacy, socio cultural barriers, traditional and religious beliefs and stigma and discrimination associated with mental disorders (Raguram et al., 1996). As has been previously noted a major barrier is difficulty in integrating mental health into primary health care. The services of primary health care workers suffer because of lack of supervision and support from specialists. Another barrier is that medical students and psychiatric residents trained in mental hospitals are hampered because of lack of exposure to community settings and lack of infrastructure for supervision in the community (Kumar, 2011). Here stepwise supervision of mental health caregivers such as primary health care physicians and psychiatric nurses by a hierarchy of experts, as in a tertiary hospital, is lacking or inadequate. If this inadequacy is significantly alleviated the need to refer cases with minimal complications to tertiary care hospitals, which are often over-burdened and far away, will be greatly diminished.

INNOVATIONS BY NON-GOVERNMENT ACTORS

Some NGOs and civil society groups have done a commendable job in providing mental health services to the community (Thara and Patel, 2010). Many have set up day care centres, half-way homes, long stay homes, counseling centres, suicide prevention centres, school mental health programmes, disaster mental health care and community based programmes for the mentally ill. Some NGOs who are doing a commendable job are Medico Pastoral Association, Bangalore; *Paripurnata*, Kolkata; SCARF and the *Baniyan*, Chennai; Richmond Fellowship Society (Bangalore, Lucknow, Delhi); *Cadabams*, Bangalore; and *Ashadeep* in Guwahati. However, most of their services are provided through extension clinics concentrated mainly in urban areas. *Nav Bharat Jagriti Kendra* is one of the few working in rural areas. It can be said that the NGOs can at best be a supplement to government agencies in providing mental health services, but they cannot be an alternative to such agencies in providing mental health services in rural areas, given the need and treatment gap as noted by various experts.

SUGGESTIONS FOR IMPROVING MENTAL HEALTH CARE

The following measures have been suggested for strengthening the rural mental health care services: 1) Convergence of National Mental Health Programme/ District Mental Health Programme under National Rural Health Mission Programme and use of existing PHCs and sub-centres to provide mental health services; 2) Capacity building of rural registered medical practitioners/primary health care doctors/ASHA workers (Accredited Social Health Activists who act as health educators and promoters in their communities) / teachers/*Aanganwadi* (centre providing care for mothers and young children in a rural area) workers through tailor made modules; 3) Advocacy through community, social and other bodies and involvement of religious leaders, teachers, local community leaders and other key stakeholders; 4) Targeted awareness programmes using available rural media; 5) Provisioning social security to the mentally ill patients; and 6) Training for caregivers and relatives .

District Mental Health Programme needs restructuring and convergence within the NRHM. The "extension clinic" approach needs to be replaced with integration of mental health services into general health services, particularly under NRHM. Involving ASHAs under NRHM is an opportunity to provide mental health services at the doorstep in rural areas. Lastly, ensuring bottom up approach and community ownership is a must to achieve universal mental health services, care and support in rural areas. There is a need to strategize and look beyond the Bellary model to empower primary care physicians and health workers to diagnose and treat psychiatric disorders in primary healthcare settings and provide an adequate legal framework to safeguard them. This has been very pertinently pointed out by Singh (2019) and other authors. Otherwise the grand vision of integrating mental health care into primary health care to achieve 'health for all' will remain an unfulfilled dream. The government and the community must come together to bridge the treatment gap.

The Indian ethos and spirituality may also play a part for a more mentally healthy India. According to some authors like Thirthalli and Jain (2009) the outcome in some diseases such as schizophrenia is often better in India and some developing countries than in the scientifically advanced West, the much more closely knit family structure in India and support of the family members is probably an important factor here. Other factors have however been cited by some.

Digital technology constitutes an exciting and promising tool. Indians have started to make good use of this tool: the web and its tentacles have spread fast to every nook and cranny of this vast and diverse country. It throws up tremendous opportunities in mental health. In this regard, VKN (Virtual Knowledge Network) under NIMHANS, Bangalore, is providing a 3-month training of medical officers to empower them in treating psychiatric disorders at the primary level. This is a step in the right direction and will be useful in expanding the outreach of modern treatment of mental disorders through capacity building of medical graduates. More of such initiatives are needed.

Digitalization is a field which needs to be tapped for its vast potential. This can be utilized for its vast reach to spread health education and help people in times of need. Inhospitable and difficult terrains of this vast country can be easily reached by this medium. The benefits of modern medicine and government help can then reach those who need it most but have previously not had any access to therapeutic means.

The ancient Indian knowledge of Yoga and mindfulness meditation (as espoused in Buddhist and other Indian practices) has been found to be beneficial in treating many mental disorders. These practices when popularised can lead to alleviation of much suffering and also reduce the costs of treatment. The ancient Indian ethos and spirituality needs to be explored for its benefits in mental health promotion and prevention of mental illnesses.

Unfortunately, mental illnesses have been previously left out of the purview of insurance coverage, an omission which has resulted in considerable damage to the financial health of patients with mental illness and their caregivers. Some legislations and schemes have recently been instituted to remedy this situation and to safeguard the rights of the mentally ill, and also provide better care. For example, the *Ayushman Bharat* (Healthy India) initiative launched in 2018 aims to provide comprehensive primary health care including health insurance coverage for non-communicable diseases, of which mental disorders are an important category. *Ayushman Bharat Pradhan Mantri Jan Arogya Yojana* (AB PM-JY) is a flagship scheme of the Indian Government's National Health Policy which aims to provide free health coverage at the secondary and tertiary levels to its poor and vulnerable population, which constitutes the bottom 40% of the total Indian population. It is the world's largest and fully state sponsored health insurance scheme. It was launched in 2018 under the aegis of Ministry of Health and Family Welfare in India.

Conclusion

Given that more than 14% of the Indian population suffers from mental illness and the suicide mortality rate is as high as 16 per 100,000, the mental health problem in India is very challenging. However, the government has reacted very well through a national mental health policy, a rights based mental health act and a mental health programme which links doorstep service to those in need of mental health care, primary health centres, community health centres, mental hospitals and other nodal centres so that every person suffering from a mental health problem gets timely attention and suitable treatment. However, problems remain, the major ones being delays in treatment due to the long distances between the mental health hospitals and other nodal centres on the one hand and entities providing services at the grassroots on the other; and the lack of qualified manpower such as psychiatrists, clinical psychologists and mental health care workers which is significant all over the country but is more serious in rural areas than in urban areas. The government should thus give top priority to programmes for infrastructure creation and human capital formation in regard to mental health care. Prevention of mental illness and promotion of mental health needs to be integrated within a public policy approach that encompasses horizontal action through different public sectors such as environment, housing, social welfare, labour and employment, education, criminal justice and human rights. This will generate a win-win situation across the sectors leading to a wide range of health, social and economic benefits.

REFERENCES

About PradhanMantri Jan ArogyaYojana (PM - /JAY). Available at http://www. Ayushman.Bharat/NationalHealthAuthority/Goi.Pmjay. gov.in. Accessed 2 March 2020.

Arvind, B.A., Gururaj, G., Loganathan, S., Amudhan, S., Varghese, M., Benegal, V., Rao, G.N., Kokane, A.M., Chavan, B.S., Dalal, P.K., Ram, D., Pathak, K., Lenin Singh, R.K., Singh, L.K., Sharma, P., Saha, P.K., Ramasubramanian, C., Mehta, R.Y. and Shibukumar, T.M., NMHS collaborators group (2019). Prevalence and socioeconomic impact of depressive disorders in India: Multisite population-based cross-sectional study. *BMJ Open* 9: e027250.

Avasthi, A., Nabhinani, N. and Grover, S. (2015). Postgraduate training in India: Agenda for Indian Psychiatric Society. In: Psychiatry in India: Training and training centres. 2ndEd. TSS Rao Ed. Mysore: *Indian Journal of* Psychiatry, 31–38.

Bloom, D.E., Cafiero, E.T., Jane-Llopis, E., Abrahams-Gessel, S., Bloom, L.R., et al. (2011). The global economic burden of non-communicable diseases. Geneva: World economic forum. Available at https://apps.who.int/medicinedocs/documents/s18806en/s 18806en.pdf. Accessed 9th October 2020.

Chadda, R. K (2015). Common mental disorders in India, In: Malhotra S. and Chakrabarti S. (editors). *Developments in psychiatry in India: Clinical, research and policy perspectives*, New Delhi: Springer; pp.77-88.

Chadda, R.K., Singh, T.B. and Ganguly, K.K. (2007). Caregiver burden and coping: A prospective study of relationship between burden and coping in caregivers of patients with schizophrenia and bipolar affective disorder. *Social Psychiatry and Psychiatric Epidemiology*, 42: 923–930.

Chadda, R.K., Singh, T.B. and Ganguli, K.K. (2010). A prospective study of relationship of caregivers' mental health with the perceived burden and coping in schizophrenia and bipolar affective disorder. *Indian Journal of Social Psychiatry*, 25: 45-51.

Chakraborty, K. (2018). District Mental Health Programme: An experience sharing from West Bengal. *Psycon*.

Chatterjee, P. (2009). Economic crisis highlights mental health issues in India. *The Lancet*, 373:1160–1161.

Comprehensive mental health action plan 2013-2020. WHO, Resolution WHA66/8.

Dandona, R., Anil Kumar, G., Dhaliwal, R.S., Naghavi, M., Vos, T., Shukla, D.K., Vijayakumar, L., Gururaj, G., Thakur, J.S., Ambekar, A., Sagar, R., Arora M., Bhardwaj D., Chakma, J.K., Dutta, E., Furtado, M., Glenn, S., Hawley, C., Johnson, S.C., Khanna, T., Kutz, M., Mountjoy-Venning, W.C., Muraleedharan, P., Rangaswamy, T., Varghese, C.M., Varghese, M., Reddy, S.K., Murray, C.J. L., Swaminathan, S., and Dandona, L. (2018). Gender differentials and state variations in suicide deaths in India: The Global Burden of Disease Study 1990 -2016. *Lancet Public Health* 3: e478–479.

DeHert, M., Cohen, D., Bobes, J., Cetkovich-Bakmas, M, Leucht, S., Ndetel, D.M., Newcomer, J.W., Uwakwe, R., Asai, I., Moller, H-S., Gautam, S., Detraux, J. and Correll, C.U. (2011). Physical illness in patients with severe mental disorders. II. Barriers to care, monitoring and treatment guidelines, plus recommendations at the system and individual level. *World* Psychiatry, 10: 138–151.

Demyttenaere. K., Bruffaerts, R., Posada-Villa, J., et al.Gasquet, I., Kovess, V., Lepine, J.P., Angermeyer, M.C., Bernert, S., deGirolamo, G., Morosini, P., Polidori, G., Kikkawa, T., Kawakami, N., Ono, Y., Takeshima, T., Uda, H., Karam, E.G., Fayyad, J.A., Karam, A.N.,

Mneimneh, Z.N., Medina-Mora, M.E., Borges, G., Lara, C., de Graaf, R., Ormel, J., Gureje, O., Shen, Y., Huang, Y., Zhang, M., Alonso, J., Haro, J.M., Vilagut, G., Bromet, E.J., Gluzman, S., Webb, C., Kessler, R.C., Merikangas, K.R., Anthony, J.C., VonKorff, M.R., Wang, P.S., Brugha, T.S., Aguilar-Gaxiola, S., Lee, S., Heeringa, S., Pennell, B-E., Zaslavsky, A.M., Ustun, T.B. and Chatterjii, S. (WHO World Mental Health Survey Consortium 2004). Prevalence, severity, and unmet need for treatment of mental disorders in the World Health Organization World Mental Health Surveys. *Journal of American Medical Association*, 29:2581–2590.

Director General of Health Services (1990). *National Mental Health Programme: A progress report* (1982- 1990), New Delhi.

Ganguli, K.K., Chaddha, R.K. and Singh, T.B (2010). Caregiver burden and coping in schizophrenia and bipolar disorder: A qualitative study. *American Journal of Psychiatric Rehabilitation*, 13: 126–142.

Global Burden of Disease Study 2013 Collaborators. (2015). Global, regional and national incidence, prevalence and years lived with disability for 301 acute and chronic diseases and injuries in 188 countries, 1990-2013: a systematic analysis for the global burden of disease study 2013. *Lancet* 6736: 1990–2013.doi:10.1016/SO140-6736(15)60692-4.

Government of India (1982). *National Mental Health Programme for India*. Ministry of Health and Family Welfare, Government of India, New Delhi.

Government of India. Child health screening and early intervention services under NRHM.2013. Available at https://www.pib.nic.in/newsite/mbErel.aspx?relid = 94602(Accessed 24th April, 2019).

Government of India. RashtriyaKishorSwasthyaKaryakram (RKSK).2014. https//www.nhp.gov.in/rashtriya-kishor-swasthya-karyakram-rksk_pg. Accessed 27th June 2019.

Grover, S., Raju, VV., Sharma, A. and Shah, R. (2019). Depression in children and adolescents: A review of Indian studies. *Indian Journal of Psychological Medicine*, 41:216–227.

Gururaj, G., Girish, N. and Isaac, M.K. (2005). *Mental, neurological and substance abuse disorders: Strategies to- wards a systems approach.* National Commission on Macroeconomics and Health Background Papers—Burden of Disease in India (New Delhi, India). Ministry of Health &Family Welfare, New Delhi.

Gururaj, G., Varghese. M., Benegal, V., Rao, G.N., Pathak, K., Singh, L.K., Mehta, R.Y., Ram, D., Shibkumar, T.M., Kokane, A., Singh, L.R.K., Chavan, B.S., Sharma, P., Ramasubramanian, C., Dalal, P.K., Saha, P.K., Deuri, S.P., Giri, A.K., Kavishvar, A.B., Sinha, V.K., Thavody. J., Chatterji, R., Akoijam, B.S., Das, S., Kashyap, A., Ragavan, V.S., Singh, S.K., Misra, R. and NMHS collaborators group. *National Mental Health Survey of India*, 2015-16: Summary. 2016. Bengaluru, National Institute of Mental Health and Neuro Sciences, *NIMHANS Publication No.128.*

Hannah, R., and Roser, M. (2020) – *Mental Health.* Available at https://ourworldindata.org/metal-health. Accessed on 9th October 2020.

Kaur, R and Pathak, R.K. (2017). Treatment gap in mental health: reflections from policy and research. *Economic and Political Weekly,* 52: 34–40.

Kumar, A. (2005). National rural health mission and mental health. *Health Action*, 18.

Kumar, A. (2011). Mental Health Services in Rural India: Challenges and Prospects. *Health*, 3: 757–761.

Meltzer, M. (2008). Mental health care in India: Pre- scribing the right policy. Pepperdine Policy Review. Available http://publicpolicy. pepperdine.edu/policy-review/2008v1/mental-health-care.htm. Accessed 9th October 2020.

Ministry of Health & Family Welfare (2014). *New Pathways New Hope: National mental health policy of India, 2014.New Delhi.* Ministry of Health and Family Welfare, Government of India.

Ministry of Health and Family Welfare, Government of India (2007). *Bulletin on rural health statistics.* Available at http://mohfw.nic.in/ Bulletin%20on%20RHS%20%20March,%202007%20%20PDF%20V ersion/Title%20Page.htm. Accessed 9th October 2020.

Ministry of Health and Family Welfare, Government of India. 2005. National Rural Health Mission (2005-2012) —Mission Document. http://mohfw.nic.in/NRHM/Documents/Mission_Document.pdf. Accessed 9th October 2020.

Mugisha, J., Abdulmalik, J., Hanlon, C., Petersen, I., Lund, C., Upadhaya, N., Ahuja, S., Shidhaye, R., Mntambo, N., Alem, A., Gureje, O., Kigozi, F. (2017). Health systems context(s) for integrating mental health into primary health care in six emerald countries: A situation analysis. *Int Journal of Mental Health* Systems, 11:7.

Murray, C.J.L, Vos, T., Lozano, R., Naghavi, M., Flaxman, AD, Michaud, C., et al. (2012). Disability-adjusted Life years (DALYs) for 291 diseases and injuries in 21 regions, 1990-2010: A systematic analysis for the global burden of disease study 2010. *Lancet*, 380:2197–223.

Murray, C.J.L. and Lopez, A.D. eds. (1996). *The global burden of disease: a comprehensive assessment of mortality and disability from disease, injuries, and risk factors in 1990 and projected to 2020.* Cambridge, MA: Harvard school of public health on behalf of the World Health Organization and the World Bank.

Murthy, R.S. (2011). Mental Health Initiatives in India (1947-2010). *The National Medical Journal of India*, 24: 98–107.

National Commission on Farmers (2006). *Serving farmers and saving farmers, fifth and final report. Government of India*, Ministry of Agriculture, Shastri Bhavan, New Delhi.

National Commission on Macroeconomics and Health Background Papers—Burden of Disease in India (New Delhi, India) (2005). Ministry of Health & Family Welfare, New Delhi. http://www.who.int/macrohealth/action/NCMH_Burden %20of%20disease_(29%20Sep%202005).pdf Accessed 9th October 2020.

Nav Bharat Jagriti Kendra (2010). Community Mental Health Programme. Available at http://www.nbjk.org/our_work/health.htm. Accessed 9th October 2020.

Pathare, S. (2011). Less than 1% of our health budget is spent on mental health. InfoChange News & Features. http://infochangeindia.org/

agenda/access-denied/less-than-1-of-our-health-budget-is-spent-on-mental-health.html. Accessed 9th October 2020.

Petersen, I., Marais, D., Abdulmalik, J., Ahuja, S., Alem, A., Chisholm, D., Egbe, C., Gureje, O., Hanlon, C., Lund, C., Shidhaye, R., Jordans, M., Kigozi, F., Mugisha, J., Upadhaya, N. and Thornicroft, G.(2017). Strengthening mental health system governance in six low- and middle-income countries in Africa and South Asia: Challenges, needs and potential strategies. *Health Policy Plan*, 32: 699–709.

Press Information Bureau, Ministry of Health and Family Welfare, Government of India. Sensitisation regarding mental illness. 2019. http://pib.nic.in/newsite/PrintRelease.aspx?relid = 188064. Accessed 22nd April 2018.

Prince, M., Patel, V., Saxena, S., Maj, M., Maselko, J. and Rahman, P. (2007). No health without mental health. *Lancet*, 370:859–877.

Raguram, R., Weiss, M.G., Channabasavanna, S.M. and Devins, G.M. (1996). Stigma, depression, and somatization in South India. *American Journal of Psychiatry*, 153: 1043–1049.

Sagar, R., Dandona, R., Gururaj, G., Dhaliwal, R.S., Singh, A., Ferrari, A., Dua, T., Ganguli, A., Varghese, M., Chakma, J.K., Kumar, G.A., Shaji, K.S., Ambekar, A., Rangaswamy, T., Vijaykumar, L., Agarwal, V., Krishnankutty R.P., Bhatia, R., Charlson, F., Chowdhary, N., Erskine, H.E., Glenn, S.D., Krish, V., Herrera, A.M.M., Mutreja, P., Odell, C.M., Pal, P.K., Prakash, S., Santomauro, D., Shukla, D.K., Singh, R. Singh, R.R. Lenin., Thakur, J.S., ThekkePurakkal, A.S., Varghese, C.M., Srinath Reddy, K., Swaminathan, S., Whiteford, H., Bekedam, H.J., Murray, C.J.L., Vos, T., andDandona, L. (2020). The burden of mental disorders across the states of India: The Global Burden of Disease Study 1990-2017. *Lancet Psychiatry*, 7:148–161. Published Online, December 23, 2019. https://doi.org/10.1016/sS2215-0366(19)30475-4. India State-Level Disease Burden Initiative Mental Disorders Collaborators.

Sagar, R., Pattanayak, R.D., Chandrasekharan, R., Chaudhury P.K., Deswal, B.S., Singh, R.K., L., Malhotra, S., Nizamie, S., H., Panchal, B., N., Sudhakar, T., P., Trivedi. J., K., Varghese, M., Prasad, J. and

Chatterjii, S. (2017). Twelve-month prevalence and treatment gap for common mental disorders: findings from a large-scale epidemiological survey in India. *Indian Journal of Psychiatry*, 59:46–55.

Sidhaye, R., Raja, A., Shrivastava, S., Murhar, V., Ramaswamy, R. and Patel, V. (2015). Challenges for transformation: A situational analysis of mental health care services in Sehore District, Madhya Pradesh. *Community Mental Health Journal*, 51: 903–912.

Singh, O.P. (2019). Insurance for mental illness: government schemes must show the way. *Indian Journal of Psychiatry*; 61: 113–114.

Srinivasa, M.R. (2017). National mental health survey of India 2015-2016. *Indian Journal of Psychiatry*, 59:21–26.

Thara, R. and Patel, V. (2010). Role of non-governmental organizations in mental health in India. *Indian Journal of Psychiatry*, 52: 389–395.

Thara, R. Padmavati, R., and Srinivasan, T. (2004). Focus on psychiatry in India. *British Journal of* Psychiatry, 184:366–373.

Thirthalli, J. and Jain, S. (2009). Better outcome of schizophrenia in India: A natural selection against severe forms? *Schizophrenia Bulletin*, 35:655–657.

WHO (2001). Atlas: Country profiles on mental health resources. World Health Organisation, Geneva. http://www.who.int/mental_health/media/en/243.pdf Accessed 9th October 2020.

WHO (2001). The World Health Report 2001. *Mental health: New understandings, new hope*. Geneva: World Health Organization.

WHO (2004). *Promoting mental health: concepts, emerging evidence, practice (Summary Report)*. Geneva: World Health Organization.

WHO (2005). Mental Health Atlas". World Health Organisation, Geneva. http://www.who.int/mental_health/evidence/atlas/global_results.pdf. Accessed 9th October 2020.

WHO (2017). World Mental Health Atlas. Geneva: World Health Organization.

World Health Organization and Calouste Gulbenkian Foundation (2014). *Social determinants of mental health*. Geneva, World Health Organization.

World Health Organization. *Promoting mental health: concepts, emerging evidence, practice (Summary Report).* Geneva: World Health Organization; 2004.[Google Scholar].

World Mental Health Atlas (2017). Geneva: World Health Organization.

In: A Socio-Economic and Demographic ...   ISBN: 978-1-53619-023-6
Editors: A. Rodriguez Andres et al.   © 2021 Nova Science Publishers, Inc.

Chapter 7

THE MALE-FEMALE RATIO OF SUICIDE RATES AS A MEASURE OF GENDER BIAS

Siddhartha Mitra[1,*], *Sangeeta Shroff*[2]
and Vanshika Agarwal[3]

[1]Department of Economics, Jadavpur University, Kolkata, India
[2]Gokhale Institute of Politics and Economics, Pune, Maharashtra, India
[3]St. Stephen's College, New Delhi, Delhi, India

ABSTRACT

This paper estimates and examines the value of the ratio of male and female suicide rates over nearly the last three decades to see how the relative 'unfreedom' or 'lack of freedom' of women has changed over time for individual territories in India, and across these territories at each point of time. Around 80% of the territories show a positive and significant growth rate of the mentioned ratio, highlighting a trend of reduced 'unfreedom' or improved status of women. There is a lot of variation in these growth rates and as a result the ranking of territories

---

[*] Corresponding Author's E-mail: mitsid@yahoo.com.

based on the mentioned ratio changes significantly from the beginning of the studied period to its end. In the end, the paper examines the significance of separate impacts of variables which, on the basis of analysis, appear to be key determinants of the mentioned ratio. The panel and pooled regressions do not add as much to our understanding of impacts as desired as these variables – male, female and overall literacy rates and per capita income – are highly correlated with each other. A regression with overall literacy rate – whose impact is a good proxy for the combined effects of female and male literacy rates – as the sole independent variable reveals its statistical significance and a one percent increase in the ratio for a percentage point change in the independent variable.

Keywords: suicide rates, panel data models, gender bias

INTRODUCTION

The causes of suicide vary across nations because of differences in the socio-economic milieu. However, various country specific studies reveal a common feature: the suicide rate among men is higher than that of women (WHO, 2016), the exceptions being Lesotho, Myanmar, China, Bangladesh, Morocco and Pakistan. The suicide rates and the male-female suicide ratios (in other words, the ratio of male and female suicide rates) also vary for countries across time because of secular changes in the socio-economic milieu with implications for the freedom and empowerment of women among other factors.

Washington University in St. Louis (1998) points out that even though the incidence of depression is higher among women than among men there are certain factors which tend to enhance the male-female suicide ratio and take it above unity. First, women tend to share their problems more with the outside world as part of a problem-solving approach. This implies that the probability of women seeking help from physicians and psychiatrists, thereby undergoing treatment, is much more. Second, the multiple roles they take on in life give them access to a greater support network for problem solving and make committing suicides unnecessary (Steen and Mayer, 2003). Third, actual suicides as a share of suicide attempts is much lower among women as suicide attempts among women are often not designed by women to actually result in suicide but to draw attention to a problem within the family. Thus, means such as sleeping pill overdose, which potentially result in a failed suicide attempt, are undertaken mostly by women. Third, women are likely to hold religious beliefs and negative attitudes towards suicides (Steen and Mayer, 2003).

Fourth, in developing countries it is men who are generally subjected to the stress and uncertainty of being breadwinners in their families. This stress drives the male suicide rate up as a multiple of the female suicide rate. However, this factor alone is surely not responsible for the significant gulf between male and female suicide rates observed across the world as in developed countries, where women rival men in regard to earning family income, male suicide rates are again distinctly higher than the female suicide rates. Nevertheless, we can use the WHO dataset mentioned above to examine whether the sharing of the mentioned burden of earning family income drives the male-female ratio of suicide rates down in developed countries as compared to developing countries. Let us compare the four large developed countries of United States, Germany, France, and Japan with the four large developing countries of China, India, Bangladesh, and Pakistan. In the four developing countries the male-female suicide ratio is 0.95, 1.28, 0.82 and 0.97 respectively. In the four developed countries the ratio is respectively 3.3, 2.83, 2.75 and 2.53. These figures tell us that in spite of sharing the stress of earning the family income, females in developed countries display a suicide rate which is a smaller multiple of the male suicide rate as compared to developing countries. An educated guess would be that there are factors characterizing developed countries such as higher literacy and better institutions which drive female empowerment up and therefore female-male (male-female) suicide ratio down (up).

In general, if we neglect differential pressures in regard to bearing the burden of earning family income on adult males and females, factors which push the freedom of women down through lower female empowerment should be the only significant ones which push the male-female suicide ratio down. Thus, male-female suicide ratio can be taken to be an index of female "unfreedom" (defined in the sense of Sen, 1999) relative to that of men which encompasses physical or sexual abuse, lack of economic opportunities etc., and lack of liberty to voice complaints about the denial of mentioned elementary freedoms. The neglect of 'differential pressures', as mentioned above, might be justified as some stress often yields more satisfaction than 'no stress'. It can be inferred, for example, from Bean and Bradley (1986), that stress presents challenges to a human which when overcome produce positive life satisfaction. Further, the income earning power of women in developed countries empowers women and brings them in greater touch with the external world. This can be seen as enhancing life satisfaction and actually bringing the male-female suicide ratio down.

Intuitively, therefore we see that the male-female suicide ratio should be a good index of the 'relative unfreedom' of women. Moreover, a casual look at gender bias across the countries of the world through case studies or indices such as representation of women in legislative bodies shows that there is significant variation in such bias. This variation is also seen in the male-female suicide ratio.

Consider the data from WHO (2016) which provides data on age adjusted male and female suicide rates for 2016. Age adjustment involves finding the national male or female suicide rate as a weighted average of the suicide rates in different age groups, the weight being the share of each age group in the WHO standard population. The highest male-female suicide ratio (MENFEM) is observed for Ukraine at 7.34. The total number of countries with a value of MENFEM greater than or equal to 6 is 14 (7.69% of 182, the total number of studied countries). As many as 36 countries (19.78%) exhibit a value of MENFEM greater than or equal to 4 and below 6, 104 (57.14%) countries exhibit a value between 2 and 4, 22 countries lie between 1 and 2 (12.09%) and only 6 countries lie below 1 (3.3%).

Thus, we see an immense variation in the male-female suicide ratio which we argue mirrors that perceived in gender bias. It must be admitted though that the variation of this ratio within a country is a better measure of the variation in gender bias than the variation of this ratio across countries in the world. This is because a component of cultural variation which has nothing to do with 'gender bias' might influence the variation of male-female suicide ratios across countries: in some cultures, boys are groomed to be 'men' by discouraging them from expressing their emotions and asking for help. Strictly speaking, this has got nothing to do with bias against women or 'gender bias' but brings about variation in male-female suicide ratios across countries: the more the culture requires men to fit the 'strong self-reliant male' stereotype, the more will be the pressure on men to bottle up their emotions and family related and economic problems confronting them, and therefore the higher will the male-female suicide ratio. It would be natural to expect that this aspect of culture will vary less within a country as compared to across countries the world over. Thus, we can expect a lion's share of the variation in the male-female suicide ratio to be solely driven by variation in gender bias.

It is important to note that it is possible to have measures of specific 'unfreedoms' such as incidence of physical violence against women, sexual abuse of women, incidence of honour killings, etc. However, there is a culture of silence which leads to the underreporting of the incidence of such unfreedoms (Kishor, 2005). Thus, not only do we encounter the problem of a lack of basis for assigning weights to these specific unfreedoms to arrive at a comprehensive index of female unfreedom relative to that of men we are also faced by underreporting leading to a downward bias in estimation of specific unfreedoms. Note that reported and unreported instances of unfreedom both have a chance of impacting the male-female suicide ratio. Thus, an aggregate measure of gender bias as captured by the suicide ratio does not suffer from the same extent of underreporting that mentioned measures based on the reporting of specific unfreedoms do. Nor can the suicide ratio be proxied by a measure based on the incidence of mental disorders. This is because suicide rates do not follow from the incidence and severity of mental disorders: even though 90% of people committing suicide have a diagnosable mental disorder at the time of death, only a small proportion of those with mental disorders actually attempt suicide and these are not necessarily people with severe mental disorders (Sher 2004). In order to trigger off a suicide attempt by a person with a mental disorder, he/she has to be subjected to one or more adverse phenomena and circumstances: loss of job, wealth and property, unemployment, history of physical or sexual abuse, etc. Each factor supplements the effect of other factors in triggering suicide and some factors such as history of physical or sexual abuse act exclusively on the female part of the adult population. In other words, the marginal effect of each factor on life satisfaction is negative (Sher, 2004; Gaynes et al., 2004). In this regard note the conclusion by Koivumaa-Honkanen et al. (2001), reached on the basis of a 20-year-old study of Finnish Twin Cohorts, that people who committed suicide were more likely to be those who obtained 'low life satisfaction'. The occurrence of each triggering factor, as listed above, would enhance the proportion of the population with 'low life satisfaction' and thus enhance suicide rates.

This paper repeats the empirical exercise in Mitra and Shroff (2008) for a more recent data set covering the period 1993-2016 and as many Indian states and union territories as possible. In the next section we discuss how data on various variables, which are relevant for our empirical exercises, are extracted or derived from various sources. The empirical exercises are as follows: First the male-female suicide ratio, a measure of gender bias as explained, is computed which enables us to rank states and union territories in the initial and final years. As the suicide ratio is a measure of gender bias, data on male-female suicide ratio helps us ascertain whether gender bias has increased/decreased in each state and union territory over the period 1993-2016 at a rate which is statistically significant. Finally, we examine whether certain potential socio-economic determinants of gender bias, such as per capita income and literacy, actually have a statistically significant impact on it.

CONSTRUCTION OF DATASET

A data panel for the years 1993, 1999, 2005, 2011 and 2016 and states and union territories of India is constructed for the following variables: male and female suicide rates, male-female suicide ratio, net state domestic product per capita, overall literacy rate, and male and female literacy rate. The years 1993, 1999, 2005, 2011 and 2016 correspond to the variable, *time,* and take the values 1, 7, 13, 19, 24.

Data on the number of male and female suicides in various states and union territories for various years is obtained from a publication series of the National Crime Records Bureau entitled *Accidental Deaths and Suicides in India* (ADSI). The male/female suicide rates – number of male/female suicides per 100,000 population– in a state/union territory (state/UT) is worked out for the mentioned years by dividing the number of male/female suicides in that state/UT by its male/female population in lakhs. For Madhya Pradesh, Bihar, Andhra Pradesh and Uttar Pradesh – which have got partitioned into two states each during the study period – we refer to the original undivided territory of the state, the unit of analysis, by using the name of the state. Thus, in any year of the study, 'Madhya Pradesh' refers to the area covered by present day Chattisgarh plus the area covered by present day Madhya Pradesh as the new state of Chattisgarh was carved out of Madhya Pradesh in 2000 (Maps of India1). Therefore, the number of suicides (overall/male/female) in 'Madhya Pradesh' in a pre-partition year is considered by us to be that listed by ADSI under the label of 'Madhya Pradesh'. However, in any year after partition, the number of suicides in 'Madhya Pradesh' would be considered by us as that reported by ADSI under the label of 'Madhya Pradesh' plus the number of suicides reported by ADSI under the label of 'Chattisgarh'. Similar practices are adopted for Uttar Pradesh and Bihar from which Uttarakhand and Jharkhand were carved out respectively in 2000 (Maps of India2, Maps of India3). Correspondingly, the same mechanism is employed for Andhra Pradesh, from which the modern-day territory of Telangana was carved out in 2014.

Data on total male and female population of Indian states/UTs used for the study is based on (a) Census population data provided in *Economic Survey 2019 -20*, brought out by Ministry of Finance (2020), for the years 1991, 2001 and 2011 and (b) data on state/UT specific sex ratio in the mentioned years published in *Women and Men in India, 2018* brought out by Ministry of Statistics and Programme Implementation, Government of

India. The figures for sex ratio and total population for the Census Years are used to generate figures for male and female population for those years. Note that the total male/female population of Madhya Pradesh, Bihar and Uttar Pradesh is listed in our data set as the sum of male/female populations of the two states that account for the undivided area of each of the states today. Based on average annual growth rate of male/female population between 1991 and 2001, data for male/female population of various states/UTs for 1993 and 1999 is generated using the year 1991 as base. A similar procedure is followed for 2005, the relevant Census years being 2001 and 2011. Data for 2016 is generated by using the Census male/female population for 2011 as base and the average annual growth for the period, 2001-2011.

Data on overall, male and female literacy rates for various states/UTs in India in Census years 1991, 2001 and 2011 has been taken from *Women and Men in India, 2014* brought out by Ministry of Statistics and Programme Implementation, Government of India. The overall/ female literacy rate n years after 1991 (2001) where $n<10$ is calculated as the sum of the overall/female literacy rate in 1991 (2001) and n times the average yearly difference in overall/female literacy rate between 2001 (2011) and 1991 (2001). The overall/female literacy rate for a year which is n years after 2011 is calculated by taking the sum of the literacy rate in 2011 and n times the average annual difference in overall/female literacy rates between 2011 and 2001. It is in this manner that we obtain the overall and female literacy rates for 1993, 1999, 2005, 2011 and 2016 with all but those for the year 2011 generated through interpolation as discussed. For the non-Census years, we account for the fact that the overall literacy rate is a weighted average of the male and female literacy rates, the weights being the share of males and females in total population. Once we insert the numbers for female and overall literacy rates in this identity, we get the numbers for male literacy rate.

In regard to the states which underwent partition in 2000 – Madhya Pradesh, Bihar and Uttar Pradesh – we calculate the overall/female/ male literacy rates for the area under the undivided states in the Census Years 1991, 2001 and 2011 as follows: a weighted average of the overall/

female/male literacy rates of the parts is taken, the weights being the shares of the overall/female/male populations of the parts in the overall/female/male population of the area under the undivided state. Having obtained the overall/female/male literacy rates for area under undivided Madhya Pradesh, Bihar and Uttar Pradesh in the Census years 1991, 2001 and 2011 we generate data for 1993, 1999, 2005, 2011 and 2016 using the method discussed in the last paragraph. Our data source reports overall/female/male literacy rates for pre-partitioned Andhra Pradesh for all the three census years – 1991, 2001 and 2011 – which are relevant for our study. Data on overall/female/male literacy rates for Andhra Pradesh for all the five years in our study period is derived from or taken from this data pertaining to the Census years. Thus, these figures correspond to the entirety of the old territory of Andhra Pradesh before partition. This is true even for the last year covered by our study, 2016 even though the partition of Andhra Pradesh to give birth to Telangana took place in 2014.

Our methodology has to be tweaked a little bit for the states of Jammu and Kashmir and Mizoram. Note that data on literacy rates (overall/female/male) are not available for Jammu and Kashmir in 1991. Thus, we use the average annual percentage point increases in overall and female literacy rates in the period 2001-11, *po* and *pf*, for calculating the overall/female literacy rates in a year which occurs after 1991 but n years before 2001 as follows: (i) overall literacy rate in 2001 less *npo,* and (ii) female literacy rate in 2001 less n*pf*. The methodology for generating data on overall/female/male literacy in the years after 2001 is the same as that stated in the paragraph before the last. In regard to Mizoram, data on the overall literacy rate is not available for 1991 and is calculated very easily as the weighted average of male and female literacy rates, the respective weights being the share of male/female population in total population.

Finally, we generate a series of net state domestic product per capita at factor cost at 1993-94 prices for years starting from 1993-94. The data source used is the *Handbook of Statistics on Indian States 2018-19* (RBI 2019). It provides data on per capita net state domestic product for the period from 1993-94 to 2016-17 for every state/UT as a time series made out of sub-series in which the sub-series are expressed at different prices.

However, because two consecutive sub-series have a year of overlap it is possible to construct a GDP deflator for each of the years after assuming the base year to be 1993-94 i.e., the value of the GDP deflator is 100 in 1993-94. This enables us to construct a series for per capita net state domestic product at factor cost for 1993, 1999, 2005, 2011 and 2016 at base year prices.

RESULTS

Table 1 shows the results of regressing log MENFEM with respect to time. Regressions for individual states and union territories have been conducted over 29 time periods, that is, from 1990 to 2018. The coefficient of time gives the annual growth rate of MENFEM. Lakshadweep has been excluded from this exercise since suicide is not a common phenomenon in the UT. Out of 28 states and union territories only three – Uttar Pradesh, Chandigarh and Meghalaya – exhibit statistically insignificant growth rates. Thus, it is only for these territories that we fail to reject the hypothesis that MENFEM is unchanged for the period under study. Of the other 25 territories, only Manipur and Nagaland depict significant and negative growth rates in MENFEM i.e., the relative unfreedom of women increases significantly. As many as 23 out of the 25 territories exhibit significant and positive growth rates in MENFEM i.e., the relative unfreedom of women declines significantly. Thus, there is a general tendency among territories to depict a lower relative unfreedom of women.

Consider the exercise conducted by Mitra and Shroff (2008) for a much earlier period, 1975-2001 and 22 states. In this case we find the two phenomena of significantly increasing relative unfreedom of women and statistically insignificant change in relative unfreedom of women to be quite widespread. In fact, no general conclusion of improvement in the status of women can be made for 1975-2001. Thus, the trend regarding relative unfreedom of women is remarkably different in this period from the period being studied by this paper. If we look at Table 1, 8 of the states show very high growth rates of MENFEM of greater than 2% per annum:

Maharashtra and Haryana show the highest growth rates of 3.30% and 3.07% respectively; and Andhra Pradesh, Gujarat, Rajasthan, Andaman and Nicobar, Delhi and Pondicherry exhibit growth rates which are between 2% and 3%. Thus, we can conclude that in the period studied by this paper not only was there a general tendency among states and UTs to experience a statistically significant reduction in gender bias, this reduction often took place at a fast rate.

Table 1. Growth Rate of MENFEM and its Significance over the Study Period

State/UT	MENFEM growth rates (%)	Statistical Significance	Relationship
Andhra Pradesh	2.57	significant at 1%	Positive
Arunachal Pradesh	0.98	significant at 10%	Positive
Assam	0.67	significant at 1%	Positive
Bihar	1.81	significant at 1%	Positive
Goa	1.44	significant at 1%	Positive
Gujarat	2.34	significant at 1%	Positive
Haryana	3.07	significant at 1%	Positive
Himachal Pradesh	0.91	significant at 5%	Positive
Jammu and Kashmir	1.26	significant at 10%	Positive
Karnataka	1.95	significant at 1%	Positive
Kerala	1.59	significant at 1%	Positive
Madhya Pradesh	1.64	significant at 1%	Positive
Maharashtra	3.30	significant at 1%	Positive
Manipur	-4.13	significant at 1%	Negative
Meghalaya	0.62	insignificant	Positive
Nagaland	-2.13	significant at 10% (rounded off)	Negative
Orissa	0.99	significant at 1% (rounded off)	Positive
Punjab	0.82	significant at 10%	Positive
Rajasthan	2.54	significant at 1%	Positive
Sikkim	1.44	significant at 10%	Positive
Tamil Nadu	1.46	significant at 1%	Positive
Tripura	1.98	significant at 1%	Positive
Uttar Pradesh	0.16	insignificant	Positive
West Bengal	1.46	significant at 1%	Positive
Andaman and Nicobar	2.44	significant at 1%	Positive
Chandigarh	0.73	insignificant	Positive
Delhi	2.34	significant at 1%	Positive
Pondicherry	2.07	significant at 1%	Positive

Table 2. Magnitude of MENFEM at the beginning and end of the study period

State/UT	MENFEM (Period 1)	MENFEM (Period 2)	RANK (Period 1)	RANK (Period 2)
Mizoram	5.1	4.82	2	1
Kerala	2.56	3.68	5	2
Pondicherry	2	3.57	7	3
Meghalaya	2.28	3.46	6	4
Punjab	2.63	3.36	4	5
Haryana	1.55	3.26	11	6
Nagaland	8.89	3.03	1	7
Maharashtra	1.25	2.79	23	8
Goa	1.9	2.73	9	9
Karnataka	1.41	2.56	17	10
Rajasthan	1.45	2.53	14	11
Sikkim	1.51	2.35	12	12
Andaman and Nicobar	1.40	2.34	18	13
Andhra Pradesh	1.38	2.33	19	14
Chandigarh	1.45	2.18	15	15
Assam	1.86	2.15	10	16
Tamil Nadu	1.47	2.05	13	17
Arunachal Pradesh	1.91	2.02	8	18
Delhi	1.04	1.96	27	19
Tripura	1.30	1.96	21	20
Bihar	1.29	1.79	22	21
Madhya Pradesh	1.23	1.78	25	22
Gujarat	0.99	1.77	30	23
Himachal Pradesh	1.12	1.69	26	24
Daman and Diu	1.23	1.67	24	25
Manipur	4.04	1.66	3	26
Dadra and Nagar Haveli	1.45	1.39	16	27
West Bengal	1.03	1.37	28	28
Uttar Pradesh	1.37	1.33	20	29
Orissa	1.03	1.14	29	30
Jammu and Kashmir	0.86	1.02	31	31

Table 2 reports the MENFEM of various states and union territories at the beginning and end of the study period that is the subject of our paper. Thus, the MENFEM of period 1 is calculated as the average of MENFEM for three years – 1990, 1991 and 1992 - whereas the MENFEM of period 2 is calculated as the average of MENFEM for 2016, 2017 and 2018.

Averages are taken because the MENFEM in a single year might not be representative of the relative status of women in the beginning or end of the study period but the result of a sudden and temporary jump in one or more of the factors determining MENFEM.

In Table 2 we see that only two territories – Jammu and Kashmir and Gujarat – exhibit a MENFEM less than 1 in period 1 i.e., a male suicide rate less than the female suicide rate. In period 2 none of the territories exhibit a MENFEM less than 1. The fourth and fifth columns in Table 2 report the ranking of states on the basis of MENFEM in period 1 and period 2 respectively: the state which exhibits the highest value of MENFEM in period 1 (2) gets the highest ranking (1), the state with the second highest value gets the second highest ranking (2) and so on. In other words, a higher rank in any period implies a lower relative unfreedom of women or a higher status of women relative to men.

The comparison of rankings yields some startling results: for example, Karnataka which had a rank of 17 in period 1 jumped to 10 in period 2 with MENFEM increasing steeply from 1.41 to 2.56; a similar jump is seen in the case of Maharashtra from 23 to 8 in rankings and in the value of MENFEM from 1.25 to 2.79. Similarly, there are other territories which exhibit a startling decline in rankings: Arunachal Pradesh which slides from 8 to 18 in rankings but without any large change in MENFEM from period 1 to period 2; and Manipur which slides from 3 to 26 in rankings along with a very large decline in MENFEM from 4.04 to 1.66.

One way of explaining the trends in MENFEM is by looking at changes in overall literacy, male literacy, female literacy and net state domestic product per capita: a higher male literacy might signal that men have greater bargaining power in the household which in turn enhances the relative unfreedom of women but it might also signal greater enlightenment among men with positive implications for the relative freedom of women; the change in female literacy is a measure of how much female empowerment in a society has increased; and an increase in net state domestic product per capita is not only a measure of how much institutions, with implications for the status of women, have improved but also of how much professional pressures on women have increased. Note that the figures for literacy rate after 2011 used by our study are generated through a process of extrapolation. Hence, we study literacy rates only in the period 1991-2011 to explain state wise trajectories in MENFEM immediately below. Moreover, because changes in literacy rates form only a part of the change in socio-economic milieu that drives the rankings in MENFEM we also study the growth in per capita state domestic product in 1993-2011.

Consider the case of Karnataka with its massive improvement in rank, as discussed. In 1991 male, female and overall literacy rates were 67.23, 44.8 and 56 percent respectively. Note that all of these are quite low with the female literacy rate being extremely low, suggesting extremely low female empowerment in society. By 2011 the levels attained by these literacy rates had become 82.5, 68.1 and 75.4 percent: the increase in female literacy in the period 1991-2011 was 23.3 percentage points whereas the increase in the male literacy rate was 15.27 percentage points and these increases implied an increase in overall literacy rate by 19.4 percentage points. Note that average annual rate of growth of net state domestic product per capita in the period 1993-2011 was 5 percent, a high rate of growth. In brief the enormous increase in female literacy rate surely explains at least part of the massive increase in MENFEM and associated improvement in rank in regard to relative unfreedom of women in Karnataka. The increase in male literacy rates is also high and so is the growth rate in net state domestic product per capita but as discussed before we are not sure about whether such growth/increase impacts MENFEM positively/negatively.

Let us look at the case of Maharashtra which also registered an impressive improvement in rank in regard to MENFEM as explained above. In 1991 the male, female and overall literacy rates were 76.67, 52.3 and 64.9 percent respectively. By 2011 these had increased to 88.25, 75.9 and 82.3 percent respectively. The increases in male, female, and overall literacy rates in the period 1991-2011 were 11.48, 23.6 and 17.4 percentage points respectively. Note that the increase in male literacy rate is not very impressive but the increase in female literacy rate is quite high. This high increase surely explains part of the increase in MENFEM and improvement in ranks in 1991-11. The growth rate of per capita NSDP at 5.1% per annum is very similar to that of Karnataka. But as we have noted, the direction in which MENFEM/Rank is moved by growth of per capita net state domestic product is ambiguous.

The reasons for improvements in the ranks of Karnataka and Maharashtra can be better appreciated if we look at territories which have not witnessed much of a change in rank as well as others which have witnessed a marked deterioration in rank. To start with let us look at the states of Nagaland (ranks of 1 and 7 in period 1 and period 2 respectively), Assam (10 and 16), and Manipur (3 and 26) respectively. In the case of Nagaland, the male, female, and overall literacy rates were 67.8, 54.8 and 61.7 percent respectively in 1991 and 82.86, 76.1 and 79.6 percent respectively in 2011. Thus, the increases in these rates in 1991-2011 were 15.06, 21.3 and 17.9 percentage points respectively. The increase in female literacy rate is quite impressive but is lower than that in Maharashtra and Karnataka. This can be part of the reason as to why Nagaland suffers a deterioration in rank whereas Maharashtra and Karnataka experience an improvement in rank. Moreover, Nagaland exhibits an average annual growth rate of net state domestic product per capita of 3.3 percent in the period 1993-2011 which is much lower than that of both Karnataka and Maharashtra. However, we do not know with certainty, as mentioned, whether a lower growth rate leads to deterioration in MENFEM and ranks.

Let us look at the case of Assam. In 1991 the male, female and overall literacy rates were 62.04, 43 and 52.9 percent respectively but by 2011 these had become 77.85, 66.3 and 72.2 respectively. The changes in these rates were 15.81, 24.3 and 19.3 percentage points respectively. The change in female literacy rate is quite impressive and slightly higher that of Maharashtra and Karnataka. It therefore does not tell us why the MENFEM rank deteriorates in the case of Assam but improves very significantly in the case of Maharashtra and Karnataka. Part of the reason could be the much lower average annual growth rate of net state domestic product per capita for the period 1993-2011 of only 2.2 percent in Assam. This could possibly be attributed to the fact that both states in question boast of a thriving Information Technology (IT) industry a sector that sees significant participation from both the male and female labour force, and consequently contributes to the higher per capita income levels in both Maharashtra and Karnataka. However, as we have noted before, in theory the impact of this growth rate on MENFEM is ambiguous. Moreover, as noted in Mitra and Shroff (2008), there could be other drivers of change in MENFEM which we have not taken care of such as the change in urbanization or 'urban population as a fraction of total population', the extent of decline in joint family structures which can be a source of support for women etc.

Now let us look at the case of Manipur. In 1991 the male, female and overall literacy rates were 71.69, 47.6 and 59.9 percent respectively. By 2001 these had climbed to 85.94, 72.4 and 79.2 respectively. Thus, the changes in these rates were 14.25, 24.8 and 19.3 percentage points very respectively. The increase in female literacy rate is slightly higher than that of Karnataka and Maharashtra. However, the rate of growth of net state domestic product per capita in 1993-2011 is 2.5 percent, much lower than that of Karnataka and Maharashtra. This markedly lower magnitude could be the reason why Manipur exhibits deterioration in MENFEM rank whereas Karnataka and Maharashtra exhibit a distinct improvement.

Thus, we can conclude that the significant deterioration, in regard to MENFEM, in the ranks of Assam, Nagaland and Manipur, as contrasted with improvement in the ranks of Maharashtra and Karnataka could possibly be a result of a much higher growth rate in net state domestic product per capita in the case of Maharashtra and Karnataka. As mentioned, faster growth in per capita income usually leads to a faster improvement in institutions as there is a positive relationship between per capita income and institutions. However, a faster growth rate could also be a source of professional pressures on women and therefore we are not sure whether the net impact of a faster growth rate on MENFEM magnitude and rank is positive or negative.

Let us now look at three territories which did not show much of a change in rankings in regard to MENFEM - Meghalaya, Goa and Sikkim. In the case of Meghalaya (ranks of 6 and 4 in periods 1 and 2 respectively) the male, female and overall literacy rates were 53.11, 44.9 and 49.1

percent respectively in 1991. By 2011 these had climbed to 75.88, 72.9 and 74.4 percent respectively. Thus, the net changes in these rates were 22.77, 28 and 25.3 percentage points respectively. The increase in female literacy rate was much more impressive than Karnataka and Maharashtra. The rate of growth of per capita net state domestic product in 1993-2011 was only 4.9% which was only slightly lower than that of Maharashtra and Rajasthan. It seems that the stagnation in ranks in the case of Meghalaya, as opposed to improvement in the case of Maharashtra and Karnataka, might be due to some other factors such as the rate of urbanization, the change in family structure etc. which have not been covered us.

In the case of Goa (rank of 9 in both period 1 and 2 respectively) the male, female, and overall literacy rates in 1991 were 83.62, 67.1 and 75.5 percent respectively. Even with these impressive initial literacy rates there was a large and significant increase of 8.98, 17.6 and 13.2 percentage points in the period, 1991-2011. The annual average growth rate of net state domestic product per capita for the period 1993-2011 was 5.8 percent, slightly higher than that of Karnataka and Maharashtra. Now let us look at the case of Sikkim which had a rank of 12 in both periods 1 and 2. In 1991 the male, female and overall literacy rates were 65.87, 46.7 and 56.9 percent respectively. By 2011 these had reached 86.57, 75.6 and 81.4 percent respectively. Thus, the changes in these rates were 20.7, 28.9 and 24.5 percentage points respectively. Though the initial rates are lower than that of Maharashtra the changes in these rates in the period 1991-2011 are much more impressive. The annual average growth rate of net state domestic product per capita for the period 1993-2011 was 8.3%, much higher than that of Maharashtra and Karnataka.

Note that all the five states (Karnataka, Maharashtra, Meghalaya, Goa, and Sikkim) exhibit a significant increase in MENFEM from period 1 to period 2 (see Table 2). However, the increases in the case of Karnataka and even Maharashtra are much larger than those of the other 3 states. In comparing the experiences of Meghalaya, Goa and Sikkim to that of Karnataka and Maharashtra, it does not seem that the more or less unchanged rank of Meghalaya and Sikkim as opposed to the greatly improved rank of Maharashtra and Karnataka can be attributed to differences in increase in female literacy rate or growth in per capita net state domestic product. In the case of Goa, the increase in female literacy rate is smaller than for Karnataka and Maharashtra but it has to be remembered that the initial literacy rate is much higher. All the four states of Meghalaya, Goa, Karnataka, and Maharashtra have similar growth rates of per capita net state domestic product in the region of 5%-6%. Only Sikkim has a much higher growth rate at 8.3%. Thus, in future researches the trajectories of variables other than literacy rates and net state domestic product per capita have to be linked credibly to MENFEM magnitudes and ranks and then studied.

Finally, we use a panel data set comprising of male-female suicide ratios, per capita incomes and overall, male and female literacy rates to examine how much the log of the male-female suicide ratio is sensitive to the other variables as well as time. The data used by us is that for the following time points: 1993, 1999, 2005, 2011 and 2016. The sources for the data as well as the mathematical operations performed by us to get the variables in the form needed by us to run regressions have already been explained.

Table 3. Results of Regressions with log MENFEM as Dependent Variable (Part 1)

Regressions	1	2	3	4	5
	Random Effects	Pooled OLS	Random Effects	Random Effects	Random Effects
Constant	0.367***	0.417***	0.352***	−0.0316	0.142
NSDP per capita	1.04E-05***	7.70E-06***	5.70E-06	5.78E-06	5.30E-06
Time			0.008*	5.46E-03	0.005
Male literacy				6.62E-03	
Female literacy				−0.002	
Overall literacy					0.003

Note: The variables listed in column 1 are independent variables in various regressions. The numbers entered into the grid are coefficients of various variables in the regressions. '***' implies significance at 15% level, '**' implies significance at 10% level and '*' implies significance at 5% level.

Regressions 1 and 2 (random effects and pooled) tell us that NSDP per capita affects MENFEM positively and significantly: in the case of a random effects approach the percentage increase in MENFEM for unit increase in NSDP per capita expressed in thousands of rupees is 1.04 whereas in the case of pooled regression it is 0.77. Regression 3 tells us that time affects MENFEM significantly and the growth rate of MENFEM is 0.8%. Regression 4 and Regression 5 do not have any statistically significant variables. Therefore, we do not discuss these regressions.

Table 4. Results of Random Effects Regressions with log MENFEM as Dependent Variable

Regressions	1	2	3	4
Constant	-0.03	-0.58*	-0.18	-0.29
Male literacy		0.014***	0.04	
Female literacy	0.009***		0.07	
Overall literacy				0.01***

Note: The variables listed in column 1 are independent variables in various regressions. The numbers entered into the grid are coefficients of various variables in the regressions. '***' implies significance at 15% level, '**' implies significance at 10% level and '*' implies significance at 5% level.

Note that there is a tendency for net state domestic product per capita and each of the literacy variables to go up with time. Thus, it probably makes sense to have just the literacy variables as independent variables in the regression, as attempted by the regressions whose results are listed in Table 4. Regression 1 shows that an increase in female literacy by 1 percentage point increases MENFEM significantly by 0.9 %. Regression 2 shows that an increase in male literacy by 1 percentage point increases MENFEM significantly by 1.4%. Note that the various indicators of literacy – female, male and overall – are all correlated with each other. Therefore, Regression 3 shows that when both male and female literacy are included as independent variables none of them turn out to be statistically significant. Given that overall literacy is an arithmetic average of male as well as female literacy, any change in either of these variables will impact overall literacy. Thus, any impact of male and female literacy on

MENFEM will register itself as a change in overall literacy and MENFEM, and therefore as a measure of the impact of overall literacy on MENFEM. Regression 4 tells us that an increase in overall literacy by 1 percentage point increases MENFEM by 1%. As an increase in overall literacy in the Indian case is associated with the changes in enlightenment of society via increase in female and male literacy, and an increase in female empowerment via increase in female literacy we can analytically argue that enhancement of overall literacy should increase MENFEM. This argument is supported by the empirical evidence generated by regression 4 of Table 4.

Conclusion

In this paper we look at how the ratio of male and female suicide rates (male-female suicide ratio) in different states of India has evolved over the period 1990-2018. We consider this ratio to be a measure of 'unfreedom' or lack of freedom of women. A higher value of this variable thus indicates lower gender bias for obvious reasons: all other things remaining constant, empowerment will push down the female suicide rate and push up the ratio; an enhancement of bargaining power of women will push up the male suicide rate and push down the female suicide rate, thus pushing up the mentioned ratio.

On comparing 1975-2001, a period studied by Mitra and Shroff (2008), to our study period we find a remarkable change in the trajectories over time exhibited by Indian territories in regard to the male-female suicide ratio: in the former period it was quite common for a state to exhibit a significant decline in the ratio over time which in turn indicated a deteriorating status of women, whereas in the latter the mentioned decline was rarely detected and most of the states and union territories actually showed a statistically significant and large increase over time, thus demonstrating an improvement in the status of women i.e., a decline in their unfreedom.

The male-female suicide ratio can also be used to rank the states and union territories in regard to gender bias i.e., the unfreedom of women. We assign territories exhibiting a higher value of the male-female suicide ratio with a higher rank – 1 being the highest rank and larger numbers depicting a progressively lower rank – and observe that many territories exhibit a large change in rank from the beginning of the study period to the end of the study period. In the beginning of the study period Nagaland, Mizoram and Manipur exhibit ranks 1, 2 and 3. By the end of the study period Mizoram climbs to 1 whereas Nagaland and Manipur drop to 7 and 26. Replacing Nagaland and Manipur in the top 3 are Kerala (rank 2) and Pondicherry (rank 3). The lowest ranked territories in the beginning of the study period are Orissa, Gujarat and Jammu and Kashmir with ranks of 29, 30 and 31 respectively. These states attain the ranks of 30, 23 and 31 respectively at the end of the study period, with Jammu and Kashmir continuing to remain at the bottom of the ladder. The newcomer in the bottom three is Uttar Pradesh with rank 29, nine places lower than the rank attained by the state at the beginning of the study period.

The volatility in rank is a result of differing growth rates in male-female suicide ratio in the study period. Consider the states of Maharashtra, Delhi, Gujarat, and Karnataka which go up 15, 8, 7 and 7 places from their ranks of 23, 27, 30 and 17 respectively at the beginning of the study period. These movements in rank correspond to statistically significant annual growth rates of the male-female suicide ratio of 3.30, 2.34, 2.34 and 1.95 percent respectively. Now consider the states of Manipur, Uttar Pradesh, Assam and Nagaland which register a marked decline in ranks of 23, 9, 6 and 6 respectively from their initial ranks of 3, 20, 10 and 1. The average annual growth rates in male-female suicide ratio are -4.13, 0.16 (statistically insignificant), 0.67 and -2.13 percent respectively. Thus, as expected, those which move up the ladder of ranks over the study period register a far higher annual growth rate of the male-female suicide ratio than those which move down the ladder.

In general, we can conclude that the situation in regard to status of women has improved over the study period. In the beginning the male-female suicide ratios corresponding to ranks 1, 5, 10, 20 and 30 are 8.89,

2.56, 1.86, 1.37 and 0.99 respectively. At the end these ranks correspond to 4.82, 3.36, 2.56, 1.96 and 1.14 respectively. Thus, the male-female suicide ratio for each of the listed ranks apart from 1 is higher for the end of the study period than it is for the beginning of the study period. This points to an improvement in the status of women during the study period. Another indicator of such improvement is the average annual growth rate of the male-female suicide ratio: out of 28 territories for which average annual growth rates of the male-female suicide ratios in the period 1990-2018 were determined through time series regressions, data for twenty-three territories revealed a statistically significant and positive growth rate.

From determining how various Indian territories rank in regard to the status of women, as revealed by the male-female suicide ratio, as well as how rapidly such status has been changing in different Indian territories, we shift to an examination of the various determinants of the relative status of women proxied by the male-female suicide ratio. Our analytical approach induces us to pick the following independent determinants of the male-female suicide ratio: female literacy rate as female literacy should be empowering and bring down the female suicide rate; male literacy rate as male literacy can be enlightening and enlightened male behavior can bring down the female suicide rate; overall literacy rate as it is a weighted average of the male and female literacy rate; net state domestic product per capita as growth in this variable is often associated with improvement in institutions which can bring down the female suicide rate.

The female literacy rate, male literacy rate and net state domestic product per capita are heavily correlated with each other as each of these variables is highly correlated with time. Thus, it becomes very difficult to include any two out of these three determinants in a regression and determine their impacts on the male-female suicide ratio. When we actually ran these regressions, the independent variables turned out to be statistically insignificant, as reported in this paper. Therefore, we ran a regression with overall literacy rate as the independent variable and male-female suicide ratio as the dependent variable because overall literacy rate is a weighted average of both female and male literacy rates and its impact on the dependent variable would capture the impact of both male and female literary rates. The regression revealed that a unit percentage point increase in overall literacy rate leads to a 1% increase in male-female suicide ratio. If we replace overall literacy rate by female (male) literacy rate in the regression the impact of a unit percentage point increase is 0.9 (1.4) percent. But again, these results are imprecise as the changes in the female literacy rate are mostly associated with changes in the male literacy rate and the precise estimation of impacts of each of these variables is dependent on there existing a substantial mass of data where change in one variable takes place without the other changing in value.

We also try to explain the change in ranks, in regard to the male-female suicide ratio, of different Indian territories over the study period on the basis of changes in overall, male and female literacy rates as well as growth in net state domestic product per capita. If we compare those which exhibit a large improvement in ranks to those which exhibit a large deterioration it seems that a higher rate of growth of state domestic per capita drives improvement as opposed to deterioration. However, those showing stability in ranks do not exhibit either a markedly lower growth rate of net state domestic product per capita or literacy rates than those showing large improvement in ranks. This tells us that it is necessary in future researches to analytically link the male-female suicide ratio to variables not included in our study and then empirically estimate the strength of these linkages.

REFERENCES

Bean, J.P. and Bradley, R.K. (1986). Untangling the satisfaction-performance relationship for college students. *The Journal of Higher Education*, 57:393–412.

Gaynes, B.N., West, S.L., Ford, C., Frame, P., Klein, J., Lohr, K.N and the U.S. Preventive Services Task Force. (2014). Screening for suicide risk in adolescents, adults, and older adults in primary care: Recommendations from the U.S. Preventive Services Task Force. *Annals of Internal Medicine*, 140:831–837.

Kishor, S. (2005). *Domestic Violence Measurement in the Demographic and Health Surveys: The History and the Challenges.* Paper presented at the Expert Group Meeting, UN Division for the Advancement of Women, Geneva, Switzerland, 11-14 April.

Koivumaa-Honkanen, H., Honkanen, R., Viinamäki, H., Heikkilä, K., Kaprio, J. and Koskenvuo, M. (2001). Life satisfaction and suicide: A 20-year follow-up study. *American Journal of Psychiatry*, 158:433–439.

Maps of India. 2013. History of Chhattisgarh. https://www.mapsofindia.com/chhattisgarh/history.html.

Maps of India. 2013. History of Uttarakhand. https://www.mapsofindia.com/uttarakhand/history.html.

Maps of India. (2017). Jharkhand. Available at https://www.mapsofindia.com/jharkhand/

Ministry of Finance, Government of India. (2020). *Economic Survey 2019-20*, Volume 20.

Ministry of Statistics and Programme Implementation, Government of India (2019a). *Women and Men in India 2014.*

Ministry of Statistics and Programme Implementation, Government of India (2019b). *Women and Men in India 2018.*

Mitra, S. and Shroff, S. (2008). What suicides reveal about gender bias. *The Journal of Socio-Economics*, 37:1713–1723.

National Crimes Records Bureau. Various Years. *Accidental Deaths and Suicides in India.* Available at https://ncrb.gov.in/accidental-deaths-suicides-india-adsi.

Reserve Bank of India (2019). *Handbook of Statistics on Indian States 2018-19.* Available at https://www.rbi.org.in/Scripts/PublicationsView.aspx?id = 18812.

Sen, A. (1999). *Development as Freedom.* Oxford: Oxford University Press.

Sher, L. (2004). Preventing suicide. *Quarterly Journal of Medicine*, 97:677–680.

Steen, D.M. and Mayer, P. (2003). Patterns of suicide by age and gender in the Indian states: A reflection of human development? *Archives of Suicide Research*, 7: 247–264.

Washington University in St. Louis. (1998). Why women are less likely than men to commit suicide. http://www.sciencedaily.com/releases/1998/11/981112075159.htm

World Health Organization. (2016). GHO | By category | Suicide rate estimates, age-standardized - Estimates by country. Available at https://apps.who.int/gho/data/node.main.MHSUICIDEASDR?lang = en[accesedon18/10/2019]

ABOUT THE EDITORS

Antonio Rodríguez Andrés
Associate Professor of Economics
Technical University of Ostrava, Ostrava, Czechia

Docent. Antonio Rodríguez Andrés is currently an Associate Professor of Economics at VŠB Technical University of Ostrava. He got a PhD in Economics at University of Southern Denmark (SDU). His research focuses on quantitative methods, applied health economics, and law and economics. He has published in international refereed journals with high impact factor such as: *Journal of Business Ethics, Health Policy, and Technological Forecasting and Social Change*. He is also currently on the international advisory board of The Economic and Labour Relations Review (ELRR).

Besides that, he has also served several accreditation committees during his academic experience (PhD committee, AACSB, EPAS). Dr. Antonio has actively participated in international conferences and symposiums as speaker as well as organizer. He has also ample teaching experience at both graduate and undergraduate level. He has been teaching at both graduate and undergraduate level several subjects within Economics, Econometrics, and Statistics. Dr Antonio has also applied for external grants from different sources: *Economic Research Forum (ERF)*, *and Forum EuroMediterraneen des Instituts de Sciences Economiques (FEMISE), and Czech National Agency (GACR).*

Siddhartha Mitra
Full Professor of Economics
Jadavpur University, Kolkata, India

Siddhartha Mitra is currently Professor of Economics at Jadavpur University, Kolkata. In his earlier appointments, he has been Director (Research), CUTS International and a Reader at the Gokhale Institute of Politics and Economics, Pune. Prof. Mitra has also taught at the University of Melbourne and Indian Statistical Institute, New Delhi.

Apart from researching in the more common fields of development economics, environmental economics, agricultural economics and economic theory he has also devoted himself to research in fields such as the economics of peace and mental health. In regard to mental health, his research focuses on the socio-economic determinants of mental health outcomes as well as the use of data relating to these outcomes to gauge the severity of certain social problems such as gender bias.

Prof. Mitra has been a prolific researcher with papers in reputed journals and edited volumes to his credit. He has served on a consultative committee to the Ministry of Environment, Government of India; conducted courses in Vietnam and Bangladesh; and presented in seminars and conferences in Australia, Europe, United States and Asia.

Prof. Mitra holds a Ph.D. and M.S. degree from the Agricultural and Resource Economics Department of the University of Maryland at College Park, USA and a Masters in Economics from the Delhi School of Economics, India.

INDEX

A

anxiety disorders, ix, 64, 108, 109, 113

C

chronic illness(es), viii, ix, 39, 40, 43, 44, 45, 46, 49, 50, 51, 52, 55
chronically ill, ix, 45, 49, 51
community health centres, x, 105, 121, 125
coronary heart disease, ix, 49, 54
counselling centers, x, 77

D

depression, ix, 1, 2, 6, 9, 10, 11, 12, 13, 14, 17, 18, 21, 22, 23, 25, 26, 40, 51, 52, 57, 65, 66, 72, 73, 77, 78, 79, 80, 81, 82, 86, 97, 98, 107, 108, 109, 113, 128, 131, 136
diabetes, ix, 16, 23, 44, 49, 51, 52, 113, 114

E

economic deprivation, viii
economic growth, vii

emotional intelligence, ix, 39, 46, 47, 48, 49, 50, 51, 52, 53, 54

F

fulfilment, vii

G

gender bias, viii, x, 136, 138, 139, 140, 145, 154, 155, 158, 162

H

happiness, v, vii, x, 17, 21, 22, 23, 24, 25, 26, 39, 40, 41, 42, 43, 44, 45, 46, 47, 48, 49, 50, 51, 52, 53, 54, 55, 85, 86, 87, 88, 89, 90, 91, 92, 93, 94, 95, 97, 98, 99, 100, 101, 102, 103
holistic, vii, 3
human capital, vii, 2, 105, 125
human right, vii, 106, 115, 126

I

illnesses, ix, 25, 45, 50, 62, 70, 110, 114, 115, 119
India, v, vi, vii, viii, ix, xi, 1, 2, 3, 7, 9, 11, 12, 13, 21, 22, 23, 24, 25, 26, 27, 28, 31, 32, 34, 35, 36, 37, 38, 39, 40, 47, 48, 52, 54, 55, 57, 59, 61, 62, 63, 64, 65, 66, 67, 68, 69, 70, 71, 72, 73, 74, 75, 76, 78, 79, 80, 81, 82, 85, 96, 100, 105, 106, 107, 108, 110, 113, 117, 119, 120, 121, 124, 125, 126, 127, 128, 129, 130, 131, 132, 135, 137, 140, 141, 142, 154, 158, 162

L

life events, ix, 2, 4, 6, 12, 13, 16, 21, 63, 65, 76
life expectancy, ix, 27, 32, 33, 35

M

medical care, x, 49, 105
meditation, ix, 50, 88, 106, 124
mental health, vii, viii, ix, x, xi, 1, 2, 3, 4, 5, 6, 8, 9, 10, 11, 12, 13, 14, 15, 18, 19, 20, 21, 22, 23, 25, 26, 48, 57, 58, 59, 62, 63, 65, 66, 67, 68, 69, 70, 71, 72, 73, 74, 75, 76, 78, 79, 83, 92, 97, 100, 105, 106, 107, 108, 109, 110, 111, 112, 113, 114, 115, 116, 117, 118, 119, 120, 121, 122, 123, 124, 125, 127, 129, 130, 131, 132, 133, 162
mental health disorders, ix, 4, 57, 59, 73, 75, 110
mental health problem, vii, viii, xi, 1, 2, 11, 12, 25, 58, 59, 63, 65, 70, 71, 74, 75, 83, 97, 105, 107, 114, 125
mental hospitals, x, 105, 117, 120, 121, 122, 125

mental illness, vii, viii, x, 2, 3, 4, 6, 14, 21, 22, 23, 25, 26, 58, 62, 63, 64, 65, 66, 70, 74, 97, 105, 106, 107, 108, 109, 114, 115, 116, 118, 121, 124, 125, 131, 132
mental well-being, vii, ix, x, 23, 106
Muslims, ix, 16, 35, 36

N

National Mental Health Survey, vii, 1, 2, 63, 81, 106, 107, 129

P

physical health, viii, 2, 5, 10, 13, 16, 18, 25, 74, 89, 111
physical security, ix
poverty, vii, 3, 11, 12, 17, 20, 22, 24, 110

R

romantic relationships, ix, 98, 102

S

safety of women, viii, 2, 5, 12, 13, 19
self-reported wellbeing, viii
social factors, viii
socio-economic circumstances, ix
substance abuse, ix, 4, 6, 57, 60, 67, 70, 73, 108, 116, 129
suicide rates, vi, ix, x, 4, 27, 28, 29, 30, 31, 35, 36, 37, 106, 135, 136, 137, 138, 139, 140, 141, 154
suicides, vii, viii, ix, x, 9, 13, 29, 66, 72, 80, 109, 136, 141, 158

U

unemployment, viii, 2, 4, 9, 10, 13, 14, 18, 21, 22, 26, 70, 121, 140
urbanization, ix, 5, 23, 25, 27, 150, 151

W

well-being, viii, 23, 25, 26, 40, 41, 48, 49, 51, 55, 58, 70, 74, 75, 86, 90, 91, 93, 94, 95, 96, 97, 98, 100, 101, 102, 103, 107, 112

Y

yoga, ix, 50, 106, 124